MEDICAL CATASTROPHE

Also by Ronald W. Dworkin

Artificial Happiness
How Karl Marx Can Save American Capitalism
The Rise of the Imperial Self

MEDICAL CATASTROPHE

Confessions of an Anesthesiologist

Ronald W. Dworkin, MD

ROWMAN & LITTLEFIELD
Lanham • Boulder • New York • London

Published by Rowman & Littlefield
A wholly owned subsidiary of The Rowman & Littlefield Publishing Group, Inc.
4501 Forbes Boulevard, Suite 200, Lanham, Maryland 20706
www.rowman.com

Unit A, Whitacre Mews, 26-34 Stannary Street, London SE11 4AB

British Library Cataloguing in Publication Information Available

Library of Congress Cataloging-in-Publication Data

Names: Dworkin, Ronald William, author.
Title: Medical catastrophe : confessions of an anesthesiologist / Ronald W. Dworkin.
Description: Lanham : Rowman & Littlefield, [2017] | Includes bibliographical references.
Identifiers: LCCN 2016031394 (print) | LCCN 2016031790 (ebook) | ISBN 9781442265752 (cloth :
    alk. paper) | ISBN 9781442265769 (electronic)
Subjects: | MESH: Medical Errors | Practice Patterns, Physicians | Interprofessional Relations |
    Physician-Patient Relations | Physician's Role | Personal Narratives
Classification: LCC R729.8 (print) | LCC R729.8 (ebook) | NLM WB 100 | DDC 610.289—dc23
LC record available at https://lccn.loc.gov/2016031394

♾ ™ The paper used in this publication meets the minimum requirements of
American National Standard for Information Sciences Permanence of Paper for
Printed Library Materials, ANSI/NISO Z39.48-1992.

Printed in the United States of America

For the doctors I have known

CONTENTS

AUTHOR'S NOTE

The cases and events in this book are true, with dialogue often verbatim, but names, dates, places, timing, and other identifying details have been altered to preserve confidentiality. All names are assigned random letters. It should also be noted that Dr. F, who appears in chapter 7, actually represents a composite of two doctors; the Dr. F who speaks Japanese is different from the Dr. F in the rest of the chapter. The patient-centered care meeting that appears in chapter 5 is a composite of two meetings on this subject. In chapter 1, the first case is a composite of two obstetrical catastrophes, one involving a breech delivery and the other a shoulder dystocia, while the subsequent meeting between attendings and residents actually arose out of a third catastrophe.

At all times, when referring to doctors, I have tried to use the plural "doctors" or "he or she," but to preserve the narrative pace and avoid wordiness, I have sometimes used the word "he" alone. No offense intended to female doctors, who now make up half of the medical profession.

ACKNOWLEDGMENTS

I would like to thank Suzanne Staszak-Silva, my editor at Rowman & Littlefield, as well as senior executive editor Jonathan Sisk for making this book project possible. I would also like to thank Professor Maria Frawley and the entire staff at the George Washington University Honors Program for opening up a new chapter in my professional life. I would like to thank Alexandra Roosevelt for coining the phrase "artificial happiness," in regard to a previous book project, as well as Grace Dworkin for suggesting the dedication for this book.

I

THE POLITICS OF A CATASTROPHE

One night in the 1980s, during my anesthesiology training, I was sitting in the doctors' lounge with the on-call obstetrics resident. He told me that a woman had just arrived on the labor and delivery floor for a probable breech (feet-first) birth. I casually asked him if he had notified his attending. He rolled his eyes, which was code among us residents for "Of course not," as his attending, like mine, expected to sleep while on call. I grinned but worried in the back of my mind about whether my night mate had the wherewithal to deliver a breech baby.

I understood his predicament. Before turning in, my attending had warned me that to call him was a sign of weakness. Yet when I gave him a few blank anesthesia records to sign in advance, for cases that might arise during the night and that in theory he would be responsible for, he demurred, joking, "I don't sign blank checks." This left me in a bad position. Calling him about a case would anger him, but if that case went awry, he could always say I had forged ahead without his permission.

The other resident left and I dozed off in my chair. I was awakened an hour later by commotion in the hall. Surprised by the unusual noise, I hurried toward the door. Someone opened the door before I got there and I heard a nurse's voice calling in a nervous shout:

"We have a breech!"

I hastened my steps and called out, "Where?"

The next moment I knocked against a nurse, who was running down the hall. "Please, here, in the OR . . ." she panted, putting her arm on my shoulder.

I followed the nurse to the entrance of the operating room. The bright overhead light glared in my face and momentarily blinded me. I shaded my eyes with my hand and scanned the operating room table. I saw the terrified face of a woman; her gown bunched up around her breasts; the legs and trunk of her baby's body hanging outside her birth canal; and finally the obstetrics resident standing between the women's spread legs, mute with astonishment, his eyes dilated. The baby's legs twitched horribly, alternately flexing and extending as if working a bicycle, their color turning the hue of metal. They stopped for a moment, then, along with the baby's trunk, shuddered convulsively.

The attending obstetrician rushed in. I put the woman to sleep, hoping the anesthetic gas would relax the uterine muscle squeezing the baby's neck, while the attending and resident went to work down below.

Eventually the team proceeded to cesarian section, but it was too late. The delivered baby lay on the bassinet, glassy-eyed, unwakeable, its hair covered with blood clots, its tiny body wrapped in a blanket and growing cold under the warm lights. The cloying smell of death and decay was already coming from it. Possessed by a bestial curiosity and that secret fear that all human beings experience before the mystery of the dead, a medical student slowly advanced toward the bassinet to see what the baby looked like. He took one glance and turned sharply away. "Lord Jesus . . ." someone sighed from a distance.

The woman woke up on the table with a dozen eyes staring at her. She lay still for a minute, still feeling the effects of anesthesia, looking around at the eyes while listening to whispers coming from different corners of the room. Disoriented, she struggled to get off the bed, her arms barely able to bear her weight. I restrained her. She tried in vain to push me off, kicking the air violently with her exposed legs. In her post-anesthetic delirium, her imagination began to conjure up incredible visions based on her greatest fears:

"Let me go! . . . Who are you? . . . Where is my husband? . . . Don't you like me? . . . Water! I'm so thirsty!"

Not another word did people say. Once turned on her side, her cheek pressed hard against the bed, the woman stopped struggling. She passed her eyes in a long, slow stare over the bassinet. "Why doesn't he . . . ?" she asked. She took in the pinched nose, the tiny dark lines underneath the vacant eyes, and the blackening face. Sensing the grim, unalleviated tragedy, she began to sob, her mouth twitching with suffering. Finding no outlet in movement, she clung tighter to my arm. She spoke a few more words, but her voice grew hollow and less defined, as if she were going farther and farther away. A nurse rushed over and lifted up the motionless bundle in the bassinet. The baby's helplessly drooping head fell in all different directions until the nurse stabilized it with her hand. Then she turned toward the wall, shielding the baby from further view. The loathsome scene of unnecessary death, the mother's groans, my frenetic eyes staring uncomprehendingly out at the world were overwhelmingly oppressive, and the medical student moved quickly toward the side door, hastening to get away from the memory of what he had seen.

When I finished work the next day, the darkness was already closing in over the city. A wind sent the clouds scurrying and tore them apart to reveal a sad-looking moon and a few meager stars. I went home and fumbled for my key under the orb's uncertain light. I drank several beers. At around nine o'clock I got out of my chair and, with a heavy, bearish swaying gait, went into the bedroom and lay down on the bed. Within seconds, I was asleep. But I slept badly that night, turning over and over, gripped by the horrible images of the previous evening.

This was a catastrophe. It is an experience that all doctors in training prepare for. Yet this catastrophe seemed totally unnecessary. I wanted to blame someone. I zeroed in on the obstetrics attending for going to bed early that night, and I argued with my anesthesiology attending about it the next day.

"That obstetrics attending should have been there from the beginning," I remarked.

"The resident should have called him," my attending shot back.

"You guys get mad if we call," I replied.

"If he needed help, then he should have called," said the attending sharply. "A doctor can't be afraid to ask for help."

He had a point. I felt myself on the defensive. "That attending didn't have to go to bed so early," I countered.

My attending fell silent. His glance became thoughtful. He was really thinking very hard about something. "They don't pay us enough to stay up all night," he answered drily. "Private practitioners make twice as much as we do."

"How much should they make?" I asked.

"They should make what I make," he replied.

"But we residents do all the work for you," I said, pressing my advantage.

My attending looked down and inconspicuously held onto the end of his little finger. Then he glared at me as if I were a worthless sort.

"Dr. Dworkin, as a resident, you will learn to eat shit and enjoy the taste of it," he snapped, before walking away.

Politics killed that baby. When I speak of politics I don't mean partisan politics, such as Republican versus Democrat, or liberal versus conservative. I mean politics on the most basic level: how people relate to each other in everyday life, and how, as a result, people think about themselves. The obstetrics attending had resented his poor pay; he went to bed early to avenge himself; the resident was too afraid to ask him for help at a crucial moment; the baby died. Politics.

I always knew I would one day see death as a physician. I did not know how I would react when I did, except to feel sad. But with this death my mind smarted with a hurt of another kind. I felt ashamed.

I also felt uneasy. I began to question whether I had entered the right profession. After all, I had gone into medicine to avoid politics, as I was not a master of *that* complicated art. Anesthesiology seemed especially suited to my tastes. Politics is about relationships, but an anesthesiologist generally works alone and supervises himself. Moreover, if a patient grows talkative or annoying, an anesthesiologist can always put that patient to sleep, which, again, makes for one person—me—working alone. Indeed, the dearth of doctor-patient conversation in anesthesiology has long attracted foreign medical graduates to the field because it makes knowledge of English superfluous. Such borderline misanthropy may seem odd in a doctor, but, as my father and grandfather, who were also doctors, often told me, there is room in medicine for all sorts of personalities. I liked science. I also wanted to do something useful. But I was not a "people person." I wanted to be left alone with my smarts and my hands to take care of patients and not to worry about what other people were thinking and feeling, other than my patient, to whom I could always give more drugs.

Two decades of practicing anesthesiology have shown me my error. Politics in medicine cannot be ignored. In fact, good medicine, *safe* medicine, turns on politics. Politics is often the decisive factor in medical catastrophes and near catastrophes. Politics can even be found lurking in catastrophes seemingly caused by a lack of vigilance, a missed detail, or an error in judgment. The breech birth catastrophe was no anomaly.

The public knows none of this. The Centers for Disease Control (CDC) collects mortality statistics for medical catastrophes. The breech birth death would have been classified as a "neonatal death secondary to complications from delivery." None of the politics would have come out. My own specialty divides patient deaths into broad categories such as "anesthetic overdose" or "difficult intubation." Again, no category for politics exists. This is because doctors do not see politics as a systemic problem, while researchers who might pick up on the trend cannot do so because of how catastrophes are reported. When a catastrophe occurs, the hospital medical staff meets to discuss it, usually in a quality assurance meeting or a root-cause analysis meeting. If the politics comes out at all, it is there. But the meeting's minutes are kept private by law so that staff can speak freely. When a doctor talks politics with his or her malpractice insurance carrier, again the discussion stays private. The state medical boards and health departments, however, get official reports sanitized of politics, while the CDC gets a number. Researchers have no way of uncovering the role of politics in catastrophes. And yet politics is invariably present. It is why I wrote this book. Patients think their lives depend solely on science and technology, or, in the case of error, on a backup system that double-checks a doctor's work. They do not. They also depend on politics.

The baby's death haunted me for several weeks. One of the hospital wards was shut down at the time, its lights turned off, with only the broad outlines of white sheets covering idle equipment visible from the main corridor. I would often pass by that ward unthinkingly, but now, with death uppermost on my mind, the scene engendered in my imagination an uncomfortable suspicion that mounds of dead bodies lay underneath those sheets. I was also worried about litigation. But a friend of mine who knew a trial lawyer allayed that fear. I was not a witness to the conversation, but my friend told me with precision what happened. My friend told the lawyer about the event. Playing with his cigarette, the lawyer said, "Nothing to worry about. The baby died." Apparently a live but brain-damaged baby risks a much higher jury award than a dead baby does. The issue was so critical that halfway through their conversation, the lawyer anxiously turned to my friend and said, "You said the baby died, right?" My friend reassured him on that point, and the lawyer fell back at ease.

A month later, ten professors and thirty residents from the obstetrics and anesthesiology departments met to discuss the case. I had expected the residents to complain about the obstetrics attending's absence after midnight. Instead, the majority of them angled for less frequent night call duty. They argued that the obstetrics resident had made a bad decision because he was tired. This was around the time of the Libby Zion case in New York, where a young woman had died in an emergency room after receiving a drug to control her shaking, which interacted with another drug (an antidepressant) already in her system to cause cardiac arrest.[1] The plaintiffs argued that the residents prescribing the drug were overworked and overtired. This was not the case in the catastrophe I was involved in—and I was there—but the issue was on everyone's mind.

An anesthesiology professor, Dr. T, opened the floor to discussion. He sat calmly on a chair with his legs crossed, his long white coat falling around his sides, looking like a gentleman's cape, even a royal one. He was an eloquent man, almost artificially so, in the way he avoided contractions in his speech and policed the residents' speech. For example, if a resident during a presentation said he had "tubed a patient," Dr. T would sternly correct him and say, "You mean you intubated the patient's trachea." His habits were cultivated, often at the expense of comfort, including the residents' comfort, as when he expected everyone attending a drug company–catered lunch to listen to the lecture before grabbing the free food. I found him pretentious, and yet in the midst of it all I was conscious that he made good on his claim to superiority. What is a gentleman doctor, let him be ever so eloquent and have so many long white coats? And yet, even with such a self-satisfied creature as Dr. T, I myself felt his gentlemanliness.

The audience hesitated. Then a beeper went off. As the resident being paged walked toward the door, he declared, "How about changing call from every third night to every fourth?" Before anyone could respond, he was out of the room. But the most difficult thing had been done: someone had spoken.

Dr. T kept his dignified bearing and said, "We can consider the possibility."

"Consider"—*what could be more ineffectual than that absurd and pitiful word?* we thought. "Why just 'consider'?" a resident shot back. "We're overworked. That's why people are making mistakes."

In a quiet, measured tone of voice, Dr. T replied, "More night call means more clinical experience."

A collective moan rose up from some of the residents. They saw that excuse as a residency program's highhanded way of justifying hundred-hour workweeks.

A complex mixture of emotions played across the professors' faces. Anger, agitation, astonishment—that was what one could read on their features at one and the same time.

Curiously, another resident defended the current system. A young man with glasses said, "Let's just do our jobs and take care of patients."

"We can't if we're overworked," another resident replied.

"You can if you really want to," the man with glasses said straightforwardly. He seemed to understand the other resident's simple secret thought, that she just wanted more time off, and his comprehension gave him confidence. It was almost as if he expected from the other resident an honest acknowledgment of her guilt.

"I do want to do it," the resident said defensively. "But every third night call is dangerous."

"Quit whining," interjected another obstetrics resident. He was a muscular young man who habitually sucked on a toothpick.

"I'm not whining!" the resident shouted back.

"Yeah, you are," said the man with the toothpick. Then he smiled and boasted, "I don't care about night call. Give me more. I want to see how much I can take."

Some of the residents cursed in disbelief. One resident whispered, "Macho bullshit." But one of the anesthesiology department leaders, Dr. S, agreed with the young man. "He's right. You want to learn medicine? Then you do cases," he announced. He spoke as if everything were predetermined and also quite clear to him—that the residents had no hope of getting what they wanted and should have no hope. Indeed, he seemed less angry about what the residents were asking for than at who was doing the asking.

Dr. S was a resolute and ruthless man. Such a personality was once necessary in medicine. Since most doctors a generation ago were by nature independent, great force was needed to weld them into a unity;

sometimes the sole criterion for the job of department chairman was being the biggest bully. Dr. S was especially hard on the residents, although his teaching methods were partly calculated. With excessive praise, inexperienced residents sometimes remain stunted in their growth, thinking that they don't have any further to go; it lulls their minds to sleep; it makes them proud and hinders a critical attitude toward their own work. Dr. S's constant carping actually helped them become better doctors. But it would be years before I understood this.

Among these conflicting opinions and voices I distinguished five parties, separated by what each believed was most important about being a doctor.

The first party consisted of the resident with glasses and three other adherents. They were earnest toilers with self-abnegating natures who went into medicine to help people. Yet there was something both attractive and repulsive in their benevolence. They expressed real kindness toward patients. They demonstrated a passionate love for children, especially sick ones, and were sorry for them all. But they exuded the aroma of sympathy for patients in the same way that men who have just been to the barber reek of cheap scent. It was too obvious. And their sympathy never bent; it sometimes stuck out and pricked like a needle from a cactus. They reproached those residents who wanted more time off to enjoy their lives.

The second party consisted of physicians who saw themselves primarily as scientists. Although the residents in this faction were still immersed in clinical training, the professors had eagerly left this dimension of medicine and now understood little of clinical practice, which partly embarrassed them, and even partly scared them, but which they also saw as a noble inability, of which they were secretly proud. Usually they were able to fix it so that someone helped them or covered for them in the operating rooms. The residents in this group wanted less frequent night call to spend more time in the lab. When they became professors that desire would merge seamlessly with a desire to stay out of the operating room altogether.

The third (and second-largest) party consisted of most of the professors and some residents, including Dr. S and the young man with the toothpick. All the members of this faction were men. They saw the doctor as a practitioner of discrete tasks, especially technical procedures, that one had to master. The more a doctor practiced them, the better he got, and so the more night call, the better. They looked upon the scientists with a secret sense of superiority and a certain pity, as if they were hopeless cases who would never get the needle in the right place. They didn't know their respective fields inside and out the way the scientists did, but they knew what was *necessary* to know.

Perhaps they were right. The real value in medicine is often in the administration of drugs or the performance of procedures. Once, in a lecture on anaphylaxis, Dr. S had told the residents, "All you have to remember is the number '0.3,'" as that was the dose of adrenalin needed to treat the condition. The arcane research controversies surrounding the subject were unimportant, he declared. In truth, when a patient is wheezing and the blood pressure is dropping from an allergic reaction, they *are* unimportant.

The doctors in this group were cocky because they were accomplished in something practical, giving them the gung-ho quality of the college fraternity. The professors saw every third night call as a doctor's rite of passage. "We did it, so why can't the young doctors?" they insisted. The residents in this faction agreed, viewing night call as a glorified form of hazing, and a welcome opportunity for real men to knock down walls with their foreheads. They saw themselves as heroes—military-style heroes.

The fourth party consisted of Dr. T and one of the obstetrics professors. They sympathized with the residents' desire for an easier call schedule but thought it imprudent. They saw every third night as a sad necessity. Doctors needed experience; it was as if God had intended the injustice of every third night call to be permanent. No residents were in this group; indeed, no resident really even understood this group. The two men exhibited a statesmanlike grandeur but also a glossy impenetrability; they seemed to want to live up to certain principles of character, but doing so made for a different reality about them. That they were privileged white men who had gone to elite schools made them antagonistic to progress and altogether unconscious of the demand for equality—including the admission of more women and minorities into medicine. Indeed, they seemed to believe that God had arranged the medical profession to be the way it was, and that they were God's emissaries on earth. But they did their work with an easy grace, and with such kind voices and pleasant manners that one almost thought they were.

The fifth, and largest, faction consisted of the vast majority of residents, including many of the female residents. Compared to the other doctors, they were of a different breed—those "who know how to live." By securing an easier call schedule for themselves, they believed they were joining in that normal, truly human condition that people should always be in. They wanted to do a good job for their patients while also taking pleasure in their own lives. There was an absence of all effort at self-glorification among them. No fussy amplification of white coats, no made-up sense of gravitas, no feigned seriousness, no attempt in their gait or speech to show superiority. As doctors in training, they were simply doing a job while occasionally thinking about what they might have for supper that evening or where they might go for the weekend.

I joined the largest faction after a quick process of elimination. I had run afoul of the resident with glasses earlier in my career. One day, as I rushed to sign out my patients to him to meet friends for dinner, he grumbled, "It seems like the whole point of medical training for you is to get out by 6 PM." I replied honestly, "Well, yes." He looked at me with a scowl. Yet I had also run afoul of the resident with the toothpick for being too attentive. Once, I had noticed that a patient scheduled for surgery had an EKG suggestive of a recent myocardial infarction. I told the team during rounds, including the resident with the toothpick, who was my senior at the time. The attending groused about having to postpone the operation until further evaluation; the resident took the toothpick out of his mouth, glared at me, and whispered, "You fucked up." By being thorough, I had thrown a monkey wrench into the surgical schedule. Henceforth, I was called "scientist" and "pointy head." And yet the scientists left me cold. An anesthesiology researcher had once berated me for giving a narcotic to a patient in pain, thereby ruining his research project by contaminating the control group. The gentleman doctors grated against my democratic instincts. The only party left to me was the largest one, clamoring for every fourth night call, which also seemed to me the most sensible.

The different parties argued back and forth. Finally, a resident asked, "Can the hospital even pay for extra residents?"

Dr. Z, the obstetrics attending who had been on call the night of the catastrophe, rose up to speak, grabbing everyone's attention. He was an elderly man, his face gray and unfriendly.

"The hospital doesn't care about your call schedule," he grumbled. "They value doctors cheap these days, at no more than the cost of a body." His spleen welled up, bringing with it all the hatred and contempt for human beings raging in the depths of his heart at that moment. "They search our bags. They treat us like dirt," he groused.

The "searches" he referred to had started several months before. Employees had been caught stealing bread and peanut butter from the lounges and toilet paper from the restrooms, and so the hospital posted security guards at each exit to check people's bags as they left. Some of the employees laughed as the guards rummaged through their miserable belongings. Others were alarmed. I was irked. When I told a guard I was a doctor, he said, "Sorry, I have to check everyone's bags." When I insisted I was a doctor, the guard smugly asked, "How do I know you're a doctor? A tie's not enough anymore. Where's your badge?" So I let him search my bag. But the older doctors were livid and refused to be searched, including Dr. Z. They felt they were being treated like common criminals. Eventually the hospital heard their protests and excluded the doctors from the searches. But the damage had been done.

"They treat doctors like dirt when they're not clinically involved," Dr. S said to his colleague. "Remember the radiology department? They didn't want to come in at 7 AM and read chest X-rays for the OR cases. So the hospital said, 'God damn it! You get out of here and we'll build our own department of radiology!' And they did."

One of the scientist doctors made a last-ditch push for every fourth night call. "I think residents should submit a peer-reviewed journal article before graduation—as a condition of graduation. A lighter call schedule would facilitate that."

"No one reads those journals," replied Dr. S, with a dismissive wave of his hand. "A good doctor practices clinical medicine. That's why I make sure nothing happens in the operating rooms without my signature. My department is in charge of the intensive care unit. We stock the emergency carts. We place IVs on the floor. We do lumbar punctures in the emergency room. I'd control the parking lot if I could. And that's how you want it. No one in the hospital even goes to the bathroom unless they ask you, because you have the key."

"What has that got to do with every fourth night call?" the female resident asked.

"Because I don't want to ask the hospital to pay for extra residents!" he barked.

Dr. S's harangue was enough to convince those residents angling for easier night call duty that they weren't going to get it. But privately I saw that I had misjudged Dr. Z. He wasn't angry about his salary. His feeling of resentment was more subtle, as during a conversation, when it is not the words spoken that offend a person but the intonation, because the intonation reveals another meaning—the hidden real meaning. Dr. Z felt disrespected as a physician. He thought he was being treated without the respect due to a doctor. And yet how much respect should a doctor expect if no one knows what a doctor is? Even we doctors didn't know. That's why we were fighting among ourselves.

Night call remained every third night as before. But across the country residents in all fields demanded better hours. They got them by the turn of the century. Residency programs that kept the old system lost applicants. Finally, in 2003, the accrediting agency for the nation's residencies capped a resident's workweek at eighty hours. The next generation of doctors wanted more time off for private life. No gentleman doctor or abusive professor could restrain so elemental a movement.

During the next month, I pondered the matter of what a doctor is. As an anesthesiologist, I had time to do so.

While a patient sleeps, an anesthesiologist sits nearby in a chair in a space bounded on three sides by the surgical drape, the anesthesia machine, and a large cart holding drugs and other equipment. Alone in his makeshift cockpit, he listens to the rhythmic clatter of surgical instruments and the incessant, irritating noise of the suction canisters. When those sounds are combined with the smoke emanating from the electrocautery and the absence of happy chatter, the operating room exudes a special kind of seriousness, as in a battlefield trench. Like the soldier, the anesthesiologist scans the world around him and waits for something bad to happen—in the anesthesiologist's case, blood loss or a drop in oxygen levels. "Good" in anesthesiology means nothing more than the absence of "bad." The best an anesthesiologist can hope for is for nothing to happen at all. Often nothing *is* happening, giving the anesthesiologist time to stare about his world and lose himself in his personal problems.

Having received a good general education in college, I imagined a doctor as someone who moved easily between science and the humanities. Both my father and my grandfather had done so, although this tended to be less true of doctors my age, which troubled me. In 1959, the English chemist and novelist C. P. Snow gave a lecture titled "The Two Cultures," in which he lamented the growing gulf between scientists and literary people. Scientists had Newton, literary people had Shakespeare, but by failing to cross over, each remained incomplete.

Sitting in my chair next to the head of my sleeping patient, I fantasized how anesthesiology might bridge the two cultures. True, the very nature of operating room work seems to preclude the anesthesiologist from excelling in life's humanistic dimensions. The anesthesiologist has to deal with facts that are more specialized and immediate, less subtle and diverse than those that confront most other doctors; they are facts that do not need an all-around intelligence to manage. Indeed, the most important trait in an anesthesiologist is not all-around intelligence but whether he or she panics during an emergency; thus, while it is hard for a great primary care doctor to be a narrow-minded person, an anesthesiologist who is narrow-minded can be a great success. But anesthesiologists *are* perceptive. They have a perceptiveness of the universal kind. Their scrutinizing gaze passes through everything it meets with equal penetration. They can guess a person's weight to within a few pounds because they are so used to calculating drug dosages by weight. By studying a patient's pallor, facial expression, pupil size, and degree of lip dryness, they can measure to a nicety a patient's feelings. Anesthesiologists also possess a rare capacity: they can recognize that critical inflection point when sickness passes into a death spiral.

But all my fantasizing came to nothing. At the bottom of my consciousness I knew my humanities days were over. Patient needs soon pulled me back into the present, and I forgot all about the subject.

A week after the meeting between the attendings and residents, as I sat in the hospital cafeteria eating my lunch, my emergency beeper sounded, telling me that a patient on one of the wards was in respiratory distress and needed to be intubated. Intubation involves putting a breathing tube in a patient's windpipe to assist his or her breathing, typically using a device called a laryngoscope, which has a metal blade with a light attached at the end of it. Once in place, the breathing tube is attached to a ventilator that forces air into the patient's lungs. While the ventilator is being readied, the anesthesiologist, nurse, or respiratory therapist manually squeezes air into the patient's lungs using an air-filled bag connected to the breathing tube.

I rushed to the patient's room. I found an elderly woman sitting upright in bed, breathing fast and looking scared. I explained to her what I would be doing: lying her body flat, numbing her throat with lidocaine, inserting a small device into her mouth, and placing a breathing tube to help her breathe. She showed little interest in what I was saying, as all her energy was directed toward getting air into her lungs. I asked the nurse to tell respiratory therapy to bring over a ventilator, then I set my instruments out on the table to make sure I had everything I needed before starting.

Within thirty seconds the patient started to tire out. Her mouth gulped at the air ineffectually. I turned my eyes to her hands lying lifelessly alongside her body and saw the nails flooding with a rosy blue. The nurse and I quickly lowered the head of the patient's bed, allowing me to get to her airway. I applied a mask to her face and tried breathing for her with an Ambu bag, but it was difficult. The woman lost consciousness. I quickly opened her mouth and, without bothering to numb her throat, swept her tongue to the left side with my laryngoscope and inserted the breathing tube into her trachea. That she did not fight me was evidence that high levels of carbon dioxide had already built up in her body, anesthetizing her.

I listened to both sides of her chest to confirm the breathing tube's position. A few minutes later she regained consciousness and began to fight against the tube. I sedated her, all while squeezing the bag to breathe for her. I impatiently asked the nurse when the ventilator would arrive. She shrugged her shoulders and said she didn't know. For the next fifteen minutes I squeezed the bag, roughly nine times a minute, approximating a normal breathing rate. I could not increase speed or decrease speed without causing a problem for the patient. The nurse darted out of the room while I committed myself to my mechanical routine.

The nurse returned to say that no ventilators were available in the hospital right now, but that one could be made ready in about an hour.

An hour! I was furious. But there was nothing I could do. No one else was around to squeeze the bag. The nurse had to take care of two other patients on the floor.

Thirty minutes passed. Anger turned to boredom. I vaguely hoped for something slightly out of the ordinary, but then quickly changed my mind, as something out of the ordinary usually means an emergency for an anesthesiologist. I began to yawn. The indifference of sleep possessed me.

Forty-five minutes . . . forty-six minutes . . . forty-seven minutes. The minutes passed on, and at the end of each one a caustic bitterness settled in my mind. I answered the question of what a doctor is. Is a doctor a caregiver? A scientist? A technician? A gentleman? A bridge between cultures?

No, a doctor is a bellows.

My answer dovetailed with uninvited memories that suddenly rushed forward into my mind. We doctors have a saying: "What do they call a person who graduates last in his or her medical school class? Answer: 'Doctor.'" The educational process regards the best doctor as not much better than the worst. Working off the principle of the least common denominator, medical schools operate on the level of the trade school to ensure that most students graduate. Students learn body parts the way mechanics learn engine parts. They learn machines to test the body the way cable repairmen learn machines to test for bad connections. These tasks do not require special creativity or any capacity for synthesis or analysis.

Bored with this education—almost insulted by it—I had quietly rebelled. During lectures I would sit in the back of the classroom and read the *New York Times*, purposely pushing the newspaper out toward the professor to let him know that nothing he said could be of any interest to me. I ignored the other medical students (although this left me feeling lonely) and studied in the main library rather than in the medical library. Later, while interviewing for internships, I met a doctor who told me how he spent his day "tricking the body": if a patient's blood pressure went up, he pushed it down; if the blood pressure went down, he pushed it up. I left the interview feeling demoralized, thinking that all my education had prepared me to be nothing more than a handyman with a tire pump. Even during residency I noticed that I, a trainee with a strong liberal arts education from an elite college, was in one room monitoring a sleeping patient, while another trainee with a communications major from a third-tier college was across the hall doing the same thing. I had taken a long, convoluted path to the same end. The notion of "doctor as bellows" did not seem that far off to me.

More than an hour after the intubation, a contrite respiratory therapist wheeled a ventilator into the patient's room. I hooked the patient's breathing tube onto the ventilator's corrugated tubing, checked to make sure the machine was delivering breaths, and left, feeling resentful. I felt particularly hurt because the real insult came from within.

Two weeks later I was back on the labor and delivery floor.

All labor and delivery floors emit a characteristic noise. To check a baby's heartbeat inside the womb, obstetricians once listened with a stethoscope. Nowadays, the laboring mother typically wears a wide belt attached to an electronic amplifier, which causes the baby's heartbeat to roar continuously around the room and through the walls. To passersby the heartbeat sounds like a strong horse galloping to its limits, its flanks sweating, its nostrils dilated, while the electrical static in the background sounds like distant gunfire. Taken together, the amplified heartbeats on a labor and delivery floor bring to mind a cavalry charge, the earth groaning heavily, crushed beneath a thousand hoofs going at full speed, afire with frenzy—the battle for life.

I saw a group of nurses huddling outside a patient's room. The room's electronic amplifier roared out a fetal heart rate slower than expected. Sometimes a belt shifts position and captures the mother's naturally slower heart rate, which sounds like a horse's trot, but until this is proven the medical staff feels great anxiety, as a fetal heart rate less than 120 beats per minute means the baby lacks oxygen. As I entered the room I saw a nurse furiously slide the Doppler over the patient's stomach. She confirmed it was the baby's heart rate. If the rate stayed low, we would have to perform an emergency cesarian section.

Fortunately, the normal galloping sound returned a minute later. But it was a shot across the bow. I warned the mother that we could have another problem later, and that we should place an epidural now, giving her not only pain relief but also an alternative route for anesthesia in case of emergency cesarian section. Going to sleep while pregnant carries some risk, I explained. The mother declined, noting that she had rods put in her spine as a teenager, for scoliosis. She didn't want a needle touching her back. In truth, rods do make placement of a spinal or epidural difficult. I let the matter drop.

Three hours later, with the woman now fully dilated and pushing, the electronic amplifier sounded another steep decline in the baby's heart rate. This time the heart rate stayed down. Suddenly the obstetrician called out, "Cord prolapse!" The umbilical cord, which delivers oxygen to the baby, had become compressed inside the mother's birth canal. All blood had stopped flowing through it. The team quickly stripped the mother of her monitors and rushed her to the operating room for an emergency cesarian section. Without umbilical blood flow the baby had nine minutes to live.

The mother was already on the operating table when I arrived. Two minutes had passed. I slapped some monitors on her body and told her we had to go to sleep. "No!" she screamed. I thought she was just venting anxiety, until I applied a black oxygen mask to her face in preparation for injecting Sodium Pentothal. She shook her head violently, trying to dodge it. "No! No!" she shouted. "I don't want to go to sleep!"

"Why?" I asked.

"I'm afraid! Leave me be! I don't want to go to sleep!" she screamed.

"But I have to put you to sleep. I don't have time to try a spinal," I said.

"No! Do you hear me? I don't want to go to sleep!" she furiously replied.

Another minute passed. The baby had only six minutes of oxygen left. I shopped for a different tone. I tried a relaxed and casual persona. I even took off my mask so that she could see me smiling. "It's no big deal. You'll just take a nap, and then you'll wake up and see your baby," I said with sugary sweetness. But I smiled with an utter lack of confidence, and my fear only fed her fear. "No!" she kept shouting. My palms now sweating, I pleaded, "Please, let me put you to sleep." The woman began to cry. Hysteria passed into sadness and regret. "No," she whimpered. "I'm afraid, I'm afraid."

Five minutes left. If only I could say the right thing! But my instincts were poor. I had relied on books to learn the art of bedside manner, and, as with all things only superficially learned, I panicked when put to the test. I racked my brain trying to think of what to say and how much to talk, how and when to look the woman in the face, and every second I grew more afraid of saying the wrong thing or more than I ought, and the more I thought, the more confused I became, and in the end I kept my mouth shut altogether.

"Put her to sleep!" roared the obstetrician, hovering over the woman's prepped abdomen, a scalpel in hand. "What are you waiting for?"

I was waiting for her consent. Did I need her consent? *Yes, otherwise it would be assault*, I thought. The woman has "rights" and "autonomy," all the words I had learned during my liberal arts education. She had said, "No," and no means no—at least in theory. If she had just given me some wiggle room, if she had just said, "Well, maybe okay . . ." then I would have slammed the Pentothal into her vein before she could have uttered a qualifier. But she didn't. *Perhaps hysteria is crowding out her reason*, I thought. If so, I could override her. Yet her fear was reasonable. I had told her before about the dangers of general anesthesia. I couldn't in good conscience say she was being irrational. So I did nothing. And yet doing nothing was doing something: I was condemning her baby to death.

Life only intensifies that which is in a person to begin with, and in this case what was intensified in me was confusion. What is a doctor? I didn't know. I might as well have tried to explain the concept of the fifth dimension. Is a doctor a technician who carries out his patient's will? Or is he a judge who knows better than his patient? I had no answer. No volume in the medical library had been titled "Nebulous."

Three minutes left. Catastrophe loomed. Suddenly, Dr. S, who was the anesthesiology attending on the labor and delivery floor that day, ran in. Without breaking stride he reached for the syringe of Pentothal. "Put the mask on the patient's face," he said in a ringing, powerful voice.

"But she refuses general anesthesia," I replied.

"Put the mask on her face," Dr. S repeated with cold determination, turning his thick neck and staring coldly at me.

I could not resist; the authoritative voice of command beat at my ear. Besides, he had already started to inject the Pentothal. Without any extra oxygen the woman would turn blue when the drug hit her brain and stopped her breathing. Dr. S had forced my hand. I was almost relieved.

The mask muffled the woman's screams. Gradually the woman surrendered to inexorable force, her cries of "No" waxing and waning as she fell into unconsciousness, and sounding like a tea kettle on low. Once she was unconscious I did protest to Dr. S—to ease my conscience. I summarized what had happened and why I had delayed. Dr. S didn't want to hear it. "Doesn't matter," he declared, after following with a dose of muscle relaxant to facilitate the intubation. "Delay and you get a bad baby."

I intubated the mother. The obstetrician cut. A floppy baby boy emerged from the woman's abdomen a minute later. The obstetrician quickly passed him over to the nurse, who roughly swaddled him to prod him to take some breaths. A minute later the baby offered up a healthy cry.

I tried again to explain my position to Dr. S. He ignored me. "It doesn't matter. You get a bad baby," he said, dismissively. I made one more attempt as he left the room, but all he said before exiting was, "You get a bad baby."

I woke the woman up thirty minutes later and wheeled her to the recovery room. She clutched her baby happily to her chest and kissed it. When I explained to her how sorry I was that we had to put her to sleep, she ignored me. "Remember, you were nervous," I reminded her. Glancing in my direction, and visibly annoyed with having to talk to me, she replied, "Yeah, it's fine." Then, shifting her attention back to her baby, she smiled and cooed, "Isn't he cute? So cute, my little one."

I had almost caused a catastrophe. I felt awful. Another attending tried to console me. He told me that it was good to make mistakes as a resident, so that I could learn from them, instead of later, in practice, when no one would be around to back me up.

True, I was only a resident at this stage. But inexperience alone was not to blame. In the years to follow I would squirm whenever replaying the scenario in my mind. Dr. S's decision had been the right one. Its basis had been simple: "You get a bad baby." But I could not say I would necessarily make the same decision in a similar case, for the law was unclear on the matter. A distraught mother who refuses general anesthesia has "rights" and "autonomy." The law calls her a rational actor. But the law also says that when a distraught mother signs the consent for an epidural, the anesthesiologist is still liable for complications, because the mother is not in her right mind when signing the consent. She is in pain and not a rational actor. Which is it? Is a distraught mother a rational actor? I do not know. Neither does the law.

Yet the contradiction is not really the law's fault. It is ultimately the doctors' fault. Their confusion about what it means to be a doctor is what invited the law into the matter in the first place. Doctors feared behaving like Dr. S. They feared being thought of as overconfident brutes. They feared their iron tenacity might be interpreted as arrogance. They feared their authority might be interpreted as oppression. They feared their confidence might be interpreted as autocratic. They feared their impetuous dash might be interpreted as insensitivity. They feared these things because they were unsure whether doctors should possess these qualities. Indeed, they didn't know what qualities a doctor should possess. At the very least, they no longer knew whether a doctor should be tenacious, arrogant, or authoritarian. So the law came in to sort out the mess, but it only caused more confusion. That the law did a poor job, however, is not the law's fault.

Herein lies the root of many medical catastrophes and near catastrophes that I was to discover over the years: In the deepest recesses of their minds, many doctors no longer know who they are. They have lost the sense of themselves. They work with nurses and other doctors, they deal with patients, more often than not these days they have employers, and in all this they don't really know where they stand. They don't how much authority they have, or, assuming they do have it, how much they should wield it. They don't want to seem paternalistic or bullying, but they do want to do what they think is right. They don't know if they should follow their own judgment or, instead, conform to some practice protocol. They don't know what about being a doctor should make them proud.

I exemplified all this. I was a textbook-smart anesthesiology resident, but I didn't know what qualities made for a good doctor. I didn't know how I should behave toward nurses, patients, or other doctors, other than to follow general rules of propriety. I didn't know whether science was more important than technique in medicine, or whether technique was more important than disposition. I didn't know if a doctor was like any other employee who deserved to be checked by security for stolen bread and toilet paper. I was walking a political tightrope, dipping my balance rod back and forth between right and left, desperate to keep my equilibrium. This made me dangerous. A doctor's whole way of thinking becomes visibly undermined without a firm sense of identity, for his or her world is ultimately balanced on that cornerstone. I would not become a safe doctor until I could say for sure what a doctor is.

This took time.

It is difficult to write honestly about what I have learned about politics and medical catastrophes during my years in practice, for politics is an ugly business. Some doctors are eager to show off the medical profession. Something about being a doctor thrills them. But they lack confidence in their pride; they fear that pride may take a fall if some bad points show up. I myself have never loved the medical profession with a lover's passion, a profession whose virtues are so many, and whose defects are obvious. An honest discussion about the medical profession poses no threat to my pride. But I do not write about medicine's bad points to expose doctors or to criticize them. On the contrary, my purpose is to help them, and their patients, by showing them who their real enemy is.

Many American doctors today feel under siege because of the changes in health care. They see no real enemy to lay their hands on, but they cannot help feel that such an enemy exists, that the enemy is invisible at their side, everywhere and at any time. That feeling gives rise to a passionate desire to argue—about government, about insurance companies, about patients—but whenever they lash out and have a debate, it is never really frank. They prefer to ignore the real issue, which beats within them and seems too shameful to discuss but is responsible for more medical catastrophes than any flawed drug regimen or half-ignored infection-control protocol, and that is that no one really knows any longer what a doctor is. Even doctors don't know.

2

IMPATIENCE AND THE URGE TO BE MACHO

A few months went by. One afternoon, in between cases, while sitting next to the operating room command center, I watched several young orderlies pass the time throwing paper balls into a distant trashcan as they talked about sports. A heavyset man sat on a plush office chair inside the command center, scheduling cases and fielding requests for the orderlies' services. Whenever a call came in, he would write out the request and place the paper in a wire holder for an orderly to pick up. He conserved his energy by rarely getting out of his chair except to eat or go to the bathroom. After several hours spent running around the hospital, some of the orderlies envied his quiet, sedentary life. So did some of the doctors.

I heard an overhead page calling for anesthesia to come to the emergency room—stat. I raced downstairs and saw commotion around one of the stalls. Forcing my way through the crowd of residents and nurses, I found sitting on a gurney an eight-year-old boy struggling to breathe, his chest wall retracting with each inspiration, his color dusky. A medical resident was trying to fit a breathing mask around the boy's face, scaring the boy and causing him to choke and sputter.

"Aspirated food. . . . Don't know what. . . . Can't see it," said the doctor. The speed of his diction exposed his agitation.

Twenty seconds later the boy collapsed against the bed. The medical resident grabbed a bag and mask, and he began furiously and mindlessly pumping air into the boy's mouth. Because of the obstruction in the boy's windpipe, none of the air made it through, although the doctor hoped it would.

"Stop!" I cried. "You're pushing air into his stomach! His belly's getting too tight for him to breathe!" I grabbed a laryngoscope and a breathing tube, pushed the doctor aside, and used my fingers to scissor open the boy's bluish lips and peer into the little throat.

I had a decision to make. If the food could not be brought up, then it had to be pushed down past the carina, where the windpipe splits into two smaller airways. The food would then go down one airway and leave the other airway open, letting the boy breathe on one lung. But the food could also shatter on its way down, blocking both airways. Then the boy would die. *Perhaps*, I thought, *I should cut open the boy's windpipe at the neck and try to grab the food?* But I had no experience doing that; by the time I got into the windpipe, the boy might be dead. Even if I could get in, the food might be sitting below my incision. I decided to push the food down.

I inserted the tube amid cries of "What are you doing!" I felt a pop as I passed the tube through the vocal cords, and then looked up at the boy's chest, which, for the first time, rose rather than collapsed on the left side during inspiration. I pulled out the tube and put the mask back on the boy's face.

The terrifying glint of blue left the boy's fingernails. Nevertheless, we had to get the boy to the operating room so the ENT surgeon could remove the food under controlled conditions. When we arrived, I told Dr. G, the ENT attending, my plan. "I'll breathe him down with anesthetic gas and intubate him. Then I'll pass a suction catheter down his stomach and suck out any air or extra food. Then I'll take the breathing tube out and give him over to you. But you have only a minute for each attempt to snare the food in his lung. In between attempts I'll have to breathe for him as well as give him some anesthetic gas through the open lung," I explained.

I pressed the black mask on the boy's face and turned up the dial on the anesthesia canister. After a minute Dr. G crowded in:

"Okay, that's enough. He's asleep. Let me start," he demanded.

"Wait a minute," I said. "Be patient. It takes longer to get someone deep on just one lung. If you start now, he'll wake up in twenty seconds and start coughing with your instruments in his throat."

Dr. G moved away and impatiently tapped his feet.

Impatience is raw material for catastrophe in medicine. Sometimes in medicine the need to act is urgent. But impatience can also have more pedestrian origins. For some doctors, time is money. Other doctors are just eager to go home.

Doctors for whom time is money want to be doing business, and they are usually speeding somewhere, trying to cram as many patients as they can into an hour, all while complaining about their office overhead or how little Medicare pays them. One anesthesia department I rotated through during my training exemplified this attitude. Each anesthesiologist in the group had certain days assigned to him when he would make most of his money for the week. The operating schedule would list all the patients for that day—including their insurance coverage—and the anesthesiologist for whom it was "money day" got first pick, choosing as many cases as he wanted and typically loading up on patients with commercial insurance. The anesthesiologist would rush around from case to case, cramming as many surgeries into the day as possible. No doctor was more impatient than an anesthesiologist on money day.

Other doctors are impatient because they want to go home. Medical practice bores them. They also think the federal government is out to get them, that patients disrespect them, and that malpractice lawyers want to break them across their knees. They come to work each day wanting to leave. Outbursts of impatience among them merely show how strained their mental powers are.

I saw an example of this during a job interview in my last year of residency. A large chalkboard hung on the wall in the lounge, listing all the anesthesiologists working that day, with those at the top leaving before those at the bottom, the position of each doctor determined according to when he or she was last on night call. When an anesthesiologist went home, his name was crossed out, putting the next anesthesiologist "on deck" and ready to be sprung. Doctors in the middle of the list felt a growing excitement as they moved closer to being relieved, and they glanced at the chalkboard every few minutes during breaks to see whether any downward movement in the line had occurred. Doctors closer to the bottom looked upon the list with quiet distress, knowing that they wouldn't be going home for hours. Each doctor dreamed of being on top of the list so he or she could go home early. Some doctors purposely put themselves on night call to grab the top position the next day; they were like men at sea piling onto a lone piece of driftwood, each man trying to save himself, one man on top but for a moment, then disappearing under-water as another man climbed on top of him. With so much attention paid to this particular wall with the chalkboard, and with so much yearning and hope associated with it, it was dubbed the Wailing Wall.

A lack of understanding between physicians is a third reason for impa-tience. As physicians grow more subspecialized, they increasingly know more about their own specialty and less about any other. When another specialist acts in a way that impedes their ability to get back to their offices or go home, they resent it because they do not understand it. They argue with the offending doctor, or simply roll their eyes and cross their arms in disgust.

Dr. G's impatience drew from the first and third reasons. To look at him, one would hardly think he was such an aggressive person, but be-neath his amiable exterior, lightning was hidden. He had once tried to push me into doing a Medicaid case to get it "out of the way" so he could get back to his more lucrative office practice. The case involved a woman with a history of asthma and a recent lower respiratory tract infection, now scheduled for tonsillectomy. The anesthesia literature at the time recommended careful consideration before putting such patients to sleep, lest an asthma attack be provoked. When I delayed the case to check the patient's white blood cell count, Dr. G erupted in a fury, noting that the ENT literature made no such recommendation. He seemed almost embar-rassed by what he perceived to be my stupidity.

I spent three minutes letting the boy inhale anesthetic gas. Out of the corner of my eye I could see Dr. G glaring at me. By the fourth minute his impatience had started to work on me like a slow poison. I began to doubt myself—after all, the boy *looked* like he was asleep—and once a doctor doubts the strength of his position, especially when confronted by an impatient colleague, he inevitably increases the scope of his doubts, and then it becomes hard for him to stop.

Dr. G moved in closer after I intubated the boy. "Wait a minute," I said. "I need to suck out his stomach." But my tone was more begging than commanding. Dr. G crowded in on me again. This time I relented twenty seconds earlier than I otherwise would have.

Right before Dr. G took over at the head of the bed, I tilted the table to the right. Dr. G grew annoyed.

"What are you doing?" he asked impatiently.

"If you grab the food, then lose hold of it halfway out, I don't want any of it falling back into his good lung and blocking it," I replied.

"Ridiculous. I've done lots of these cases and that's never happened," boasted Dr. G, as he rolled the table back to level. "The tilt just makes things that much harder for me," he added.

The more I tried to explain to Dr. G my reasons for tilting the table, the more I felt as though my explanation was a pack of lies, although I was telling the simple truth. Dr. G cross-questioned me and demanded specific evidence. "Have you ever seen a case where this has happened?" he demanded, puffing up his chest theatrically. "No, I haven't," I replied meekly. "You're getting in a panic over nothing," insisted Dr. G. "Well, I don't know . . ." I squeaked. Finally, losing patience, Dr. G shrugged and said something rude and personal: "Dworkin, you're a real Chicken Little."

I said nothing.

I had become quite unrecognizable in a very short time. It is a dangerous moment for patients. A doctor is full of confidence and vigor; suddenly his right hand loses its cunning; his tongue sticks in his mouth every time he has to utter a decision; his eyes lose their luster and are no longer able to sway his coworkers; his knack for guessing the right move is irretrievably lost. The doctor knows all this, and yet, in spite of it, he feels unable to change course. Why?

To stand up to a colleague, doctors must have something inside themselves besides what is instilled in them through professional training. It is one thing to hold the line against another doctor on the basis of science—for example, by invoking the rate of anesthetic induction on one lung. It is another thing to fret about an obscure event that has been reported only a few times before in the medical literature. Doctors risk becoming the butt of jokes if they sound too many warning bells about rare events or diseases that theoretically *might* occur. They are accused of "chasing zebras." Nevertheless, zebras do exist. Sometimes a doctor must insist that a zebra does, in fact, lurk nearby. But to do so a doctor needs natural inner strength. No scientific equation can fortify a doctor when he or she declares the imminent presence of a zebra. A doctor needs natural determination and a backbone—something that I lacked in those days.

I also let Dr. G have his way because I wanted to prove to him that I was no Chicken Little. The desire to be macho exists to some degree in every man, but it is especially prominent in doctors like Dr. G, who pride themselves on being tough guys and adventurers. These doctors know that medicine has changed over the years, but how It has changed has affected their imaginations in a strange way. As medicine grows more rule bound and protocol oriented, these doctors feel cribbed and confined; they long to flout established guidelines, to become pioneers and travel the open highway once again. For them, rules and protocols are for nurses—medicine's version of the prudent and cautious middle class. It is not the physician of the past who serves as an invariable reference point for these swashbucklers but the frontiersman—hence, these doctors are often called "cowboys." They love danger; they love the thrill of taking risks. Their risk taking is really quite cowardly, for the real risk is to the patient. Tell them afterward that they were trusting to luck and they will laugh, "We got away with it," reflecting a desire on their part to be seen as adorably reckless cowboys.

Few things are more dangerous in medicine than a cowboy eager to get back to his office or go home. An impatient cowboy must be resisted at all costs. But I didn't resist. I didn't like confrontation, and I didn't like being called a chicken.

Dr. G positioned himself at the head of the table. I removed the boy's breathing tube. Dr. G reached into the airway with a long instrument, grabbed the morsel of food, which turned out to be a peanut, and pulled. At about the level of the boy's vocal cords the peanut shattered into two pieces and fell back, blocking both airways. Dr. G tried to extract one of the pieces but failed. He quickly removed his instrument to let me ventilate the boy with bag and mask, but the boy's lungs were now totally obstructed on both sides.

I was furious with myself. Then, as the boy's lips turned blue, fear sucked at my heart. The peanut was choking the boy's little life.

I pressed the mask against the boy's face to create a tighter seal, but the air I squeezed in with my right hand simply went into the boy's stomach. I kept squeezing the bag, until sense and experience howled inside my mind, prodding the blood in my brain to start moving again and do something different. I thought about looking into the boy's throat with my laryngoscope to snare some of the food; yet I knew this was pointless, as the food was below the vocal cords and beyond the level of conventional vision. I was out of options. I hurriedly gave the airway back to the Dr. G and told him that mask ventilation was futile. We had to clear the boy's airway below the vocal cords.

Dr. G threw back the boy's head with all the force and resolution of a man desperate to exonerate himself from a charge of murder. He jammed the snare into the boy's throat with his shaking hand.

"Jesus Christ!" the cowboy shouted. "Jesus fuckin' Christ!"

Hope lay in extracting some of the peanut and nowhere else. Dr. G worked furiously, scraping, grabbing, and poking, each time realizing mournfully that he had not carried out his intention.

The boy's arms lay flung out on armboards, his palms, now gray like marble, turned upward and open, as if they were begging. I ordered the nurse to retrieve the saw so that we could cut open the boy's chest and slice open the delicate airways to remove the bits of peanut under direct vision—a horrible and likely futile maneuver, as the boy would probably suffer irreparable brain damage by the time we got in. I tore off the drape and exposed the white chest skin suffused with the color of lilac. I imagined the cabbage-like scrunch of the rending bone that the saw would produce as it cut through and felt lightheaded.

The whole room was infected by a capitulatory mood. Then, through sheer luck, Dr. G removed a piece of peanut. Five seconds later I violently pressed the mask against the boy's face and ventilated one lung. The boy pinked up, the warm color coming across his face like the feeble light of dawn after a long, dark night. Two minutes later I handed the airway back to the surgeon, who calmly removed the second piece of nut, this time with the table tilted to one side.

I glanced around the room, dazed and restive, my pupils dilated. Instruments scattered on the floor were coated with blood and sputum. I looked at them with respect and thanks, as though they were the real soldiers, dead on the field, deserving of medals for big deeds, for heroism. The nurse asked me something, but her words failed to penetrate my consciousness. The nurse asked me again, "How long before the boy wakes up?" I gazed at her, my eyes still aflame with the light of battle, but said nothing.

The nurse called the recovery room to say the patient would be coming out soon. Without emotion she gave the nurse on the other end of the line the name of the procedure: "removal of foreign body from trachea."

She noted that general anesthesia had been used and also that the patient had an intravenous.

And what had really happened? Two doctors had clashed in a contest of egos, with a fair-haired young boy bruised and battered in the process, until the breath of death was in the air, at which point both doctors, mortally terrified, and feeling the pinching chill of malpractice, worked together and luckily saved the situation. They finished with their arms as heavy as lead, despising themselves.

And they called it the third case of the day.

We wheeled the young boy past the clerk encaged in the command center. At that moment I had a terrible longing to be like him, relaxed and comfortable, neither terrifying to other people nor afraid himself, going home every day with a clean conscience and unaware that what he did for a living never needed to be done by anybody.

"You did a good job in the emergency room. Why did you listen to that surgeon?" I asked myself.

But what is done is done. A doctor learns early on that life flows only one way and in one groove. After he or she makes a medical decision, the roads not taken, like innumerable streams breaking off from the main current, flow on visibly for some distance and scatter over the plain of existence. It is even possible to imagine heading back, choosing one of those streams, and following its winding course. But over time the streams dwindle into rivulets, and the doctor realizes that only one channel of life, the channel forged by his or her decision, flows richly and fully. Eventually the rivulets, tiny symbols of what might have been, dry up altogether.

How could this near catastrophe have been averted? It is tempting to blame Dr. G's impatience, especially since impatience in health care seems to be on the rise. Some primary care doctors today, for example, are forced to restrict their patient visits to eleven minutes. [1] Surgery shows a similar trend. A community hospital's surgical schedule in the 1960s often had large gaps between cases. Today, cases are stacked tightly, with fifteen-minute turnover time. The rush even penetrates anesthesia research, as most recent advances have been time-saving ones—for example, new anesthetic gases that exit the body quickly, allowing for faster wake-up, and non-narcotic pain substitutes that shorten recovery room time, thereby improving efficiency at that end of the assembly line.

Overspecialization has also increased, fostering physician impatience in a second way. Theoretically, a medical degree lets doctors practice any medical field. Doctors stay in their own specialties today because they can't get the necessary malpractice insurance coverage. Still, as late as the 1980s, it was not uncommon for doctors to cross over—for example, ENT surgeons to practice a little general surgery, or obstetricians to practice a little anesthesiology. Not only does this no longer happen, but within the specialties themselves doctors also increasingly confine themselves to a narrow slice of activity. The rarefied concerns of one group of doctors inevitably become foreign to another. This makes doctors impatient with one another.

Yet impatience is simply a factor to be reckoned with in human affairs. To prevent a catastrophe, a doctor must confront impatience head on. I had failed to do this with Dr. G.

Some people in medicine pin their hopes on less confrontational approaches. A few hospitals, for example, mount traffic lights on their walls to police against rude behavior. The green light registers when people nearby talk in normal conversational voices; raised voices trigger the orange light; the red light flashes with frank yelling, warning the aggressor to back off. Yet the red light doesn't solve the impatient doctor problem. An impatient doctor can cut corners or call someone a "chicken" in a normal conversational tone as well as in a loud voice. There are soft-spoken cowboys.

Another innovation designed to do everything but confront the impatient doctor head on is the "time-out." During a time-out, hospital personnel stop what they are doing and go through a safety checklist. The time-out does a good job of making sure the surgical site is correct, or that antibiotics have been given prior to the start of a procedure. But the time-out is useless as a check on an impatient cowboy who wants to get back to his office or go home.

In theory, a cowboy's reckless behavior should be flushed out at the end of the time-out, when the nurse gets to the question—first posed to the surgeon, and then to the anesthesiologist—"Do you have any general concerns?" It is the moment when the sensible doctor might tell the impatient doctor that the risks being taken are too great, and that a different path should be taken. Yet the response to this question is uniformly silence, or, at most, "No." Indeed, at no time have I ever heard a surgeon respond in the affirmative to this question, nor have I, the anesthesiologist, ever done so; nor has any surgeon or anesthesiologist I know ever done so. About minor concerns we remain silent, as announcing them accomplishes nothing but make everyone in the operating room uneasy. In regard to major concerns, the surgeon and I will have already discussed them in advance, before the time-out, so there is no reason to air them again. If a passive doctor fails to stand up to an impatient doctor when discussing them—that is, if he hasn't already pushed back in private—he is even less likely do so during a very public time-out. If he does, he is simply telling the operating room that he was too spineless to voice his concerns at the appropriate time, when he was one-on-one with the surgeon, or that he voiced his concerns but failed to carry his point, in which case now he was being sour grapes and a tattletale.

In medicine, war is sometimes necessary. A doctor must learn to fight. He or she must accept the risk of being bloodied in that fight, being called bad things, and having another doctor hate him or her as a consequence. Even stalemate is safer than compromise with an impatient cowboy. Two doctors fight one another, but they still need each other; each needs the skills the other lacks. If a doctor cannot win a war, he or she can at least stand firm and do nothing. For example, an anesthesiologist may not carry the day with a cowboy surgeon, but he or she does not have to start the anesthetic.

So long as the medical profession downplays the problem of the impatient cowboy, catastrophes will continue to happen along this front. Medical training programs tend to look at conflict as an unnatural state of affairs, or, when conflict does occur, something to be peacefully resolved. This is wrong thinking. Conflict is a part of nature.

A medical school dean once told me that he preferred students who were the sons and daughters of delicatessen owners rather than of academics. Delicatessen owners, he observed, have street smarts, gumption, and an understanding that life is one long fight, qualities they often pass on to their children. Academics, however, live in environments where conflict is rare and scary, and where life is easy because others before them already fought for their better life. Familiar with hard reality, the children of delicatessen owners are more likely to stand up to cowboys, he said, while the children of academics are more likely to shrink when confronted with the darker and cruder sides of life.

We arrived in the recovery room. Upon discovering it was full and unable to accept new patients, Dr. G, already in a bad mood to begin with, flew into a temper. "What do you mean there's no spot? I've got three more cases!" he shouted.

The room shivered in fear. Nurses darted around frantically like bats around a house, trying to prove how busy they were and how the crunch had been unavoidable. With no one volunteering to take responsibility, Dr. G raged. Housekeepers leaning on their mops gathered around the entrance to see what the ruckus was all about. Several residents came by, bunching together out of safety, as if they were in the proximity of a dangerous animal.

Even the clerk in the command center wandered over from his comfortable chair to see what was happening. He wore surgical scrubs adorned with several badges. He looked like a doctor. But he was not a doctor. When Dr. G glared at him and demanded, "What are you looking at?" the clerk scurried back to the safety of his cage.

By the time the nurses had found an open spot, the boy was awake and thrashing about—so much that he pulled out his intravenous line. I wanted to put a new one in. Although the boy was breathing comfortably, I feared pulmonary complications later on, as repeated surgical manipulations can injure an airway, while peanuts can provoke an intense inflammatory response in the lung. I thought having an intravenous in place would be safer. But putting an intravenous in an awake and unhappy eight-year-old is a hellish maneuver that requires numerous staff members to hold the child down. Dr. G eyed the two ENT residents on his team. Both looked doubtful and resistant, and eager to avoid hard work. Since he wouldn't have to deal with any airway complications in the recovery room (I would), Dr. G waved his hand dismissively and said, "Don't worry about it. The child doesn't need it." The two residents sighed with relief.

But this time—this time—there would be conflict. "No, he needs an IV," I explained. "And he's going to get one." My response was simple, straightforward, uncomplicated, and honest. Dr. G glared at me. Another test of wills loomed. But this time he sensed I was not my usual submissive self, and rather than challenge me, he walked away. It was not a formal surrender, but when compared with events in the operating room, it's as if I had twisted his arm behind his back until he fell on his knees.

One of the residents rolled his eyes and called me a "jerk" while holding down the child's arms. He complained about having to get back to his clinic. The other resident shook his head while holding onto the child's legs, calling the whole thing unnecessary. I had made myself a terrible nuisance. But while they disapproved of my decision, they did not refuse me the right to have it carried out. I was unbiased and without self-interest; my honesty in assigning the task could not be questioned. These elementary virtues made me powerful.

People sometimes say doctors act like dictators. They do so to criticize doctors. But a dictator gains power through being frugal and incorruptible. This is a quality in a dictator that is also vital in a doctor. The doctor must inspire the respect of his or her colleagues; if he or she cannot, there will be doubts and conspiracies. If the other residents had sensed that I wanted the intravenous simply to bill for it or to go home early, they would have thrown more obstructions in my path. Because my motives were worthy of respect, they did not.

Impatience is a form of stupidity, but typically it is a form of normal stupidity. Dr. G's impatience was an example of normal stupidity. After all, most people would prefer to earn more money or go home if they could. I certainly would. A doctor must resist such impatience. At the same time, he or she must do so patiently, so long as it is normal stupidity. A doctor must take name calling, eye rolling, and hostile body language into account, and rather than complain about them or opine that people should be without such faults, he or she must accept them. A doctor's job is to make use of the people he or she works with—as they are and not as they ought to be.

A doctor who pushes back against normal stupidity should never imagine that he or she does so for the last time. Stupidity never ends. A doctor meets someone like Dr. G every day, perhaps twice a day. He or she must know that firmness never brings lasting results and that it must be recommenced every morning.

Medical practice is a dynamic process. Good medicine does not always come pre-packaged; it also arises when one doctor pushes back against another, producing a stable equilibrium. On a good day, a cowboy doctor will thank the other doctor for helping to guide things onto a safer plane. On a bad day, the cowboy doctor will shout and scream and call the other doctor names. But that goes with the business. A person cannot be a doctor unless he or she can endure being called an "asshole" several times a week.

3

THE TRAP OF OVERSPECIALIZATION

Life in the hospital continued in its inviolable order. The scene was no different from what it had been several months before. A hospital does not experience seasons. Doctors and nurses wear scrubs all year round, and the smell of alcohol is everlasting; even the flowers in the waiting room are replaced fully sprouted. The great transition in a hospital is not from season to season but from day to night.

This transition heralds an important psychological change. During the day an anesthesiologist rarely experiences a feeling of isolation because he knows other anesthesiologists are around to help him if he gets into trouble. Indeed, during a crisis, anesthesiologists swarm like bees. But at night, when he becomes the on-call anesthesiologist covering the entire hospital, the anesthesiologist is now completely alone, no matter how much fellowship he enjoyed earlier that day, and this has a marked effect on him. Sometimes he grows afraid. When putting a sick patient to sleep, his hands move as they did earlier that day, but sometimes they no longer seem to fully belong to him; they shake with a fine tremor and grow sweaty, as if disease were taking both him and the patient.

Dr. C, my attending, was such a person. During the day he worked in the urological or orthopedic suites. This had not been his plan—he had trained in neuroanesthesia—but the department had been top-heavy with specialists when he was hired. Better to let a few people do neuroanesthesia all the time, and get good at it, while others do something else and get good at that, the thinking ran. Dr. C soon found himself handling mostly cystoscopies and knee replacements. He became expert at spinal and epidural anesthesia, as these were the most common anesthetics used in such cases. Gradually his other skills faded. When he noticed this happening he fought to get into the other operating rooms, to rescue himself, but at a critical inflection point he realized that his skills were beyond saving, and he fought to stay out of those rooms. The department happily obliged him during the day, but at nights, when on call, he still had to function as a generalist, which scared him. Any case might walk through the door at night. Whenever the on-call resident presented him with a case in the evening, invariably the first question Dr. C asked, even before hearing the details, was "Can we do a spinal?" It came almost as a surprise to him that some emergencies had nothing to do with bladders or knees, and that patients had illnesses requiring general anesthesia. At such moments he would slouch in his chair and rub his forehead with his hand, as though he had a headache.

Dr. C was a victim of occupational specialization, a well-established trend in American medicine that has intensified over the last few decades. In 1923, 11 percent of American doctors were specialists; in 1963, the number was 72 percent; by 1977, it was 87 percent.[1] Today, the general practitioner no longer even exists. What we call "primary care doctors," including internists and pediatricians, were considered specialists a half-century ago. In the 1980s, rapid subspecialization took the trend to the next level—for example, internists focusing on cardiology or gastroenterology, or OB/GYNs focusing on infertility or medical genetics. In the 1990s, "sub-subspecialization" picked up steam as doctors confined themselves to a particular skill within their subspecialty—for example, gastroenterologists who worked only on food allergies, or cardiologists who worked only on heart failure. Although the literature says subspecialists and sub-subspecialists usually keep a hand in general practice, my own experience tells me this is less so now. To maintain income, solo subspecialists *do* need to keep a hand in other areas—but doctors are now less likely to be in solo practice. In the last eight years the proportion of doctors in solo practice has dropped from 62 to 35 percent.[2] As employees of large organizations, on salary, these doctors function more like line workers with a special technical skill. The problem, of course, comes when a line worker must suddenly become a generalist again, on nights, weekends, and holidays.

On this particular evening a two-year-old girl had been mauled by a dog, resulting in several deep wounds to her leg that had to be washed out and sutured. When I told Dr. C about the situation, he froze. Of all the cases that struck fear in his heart, none did so more than pediatric cases, as he had not put a child to sleep in more than ten years. Very quickly his fear infected me, for up to that point in my training I had done only a handful of cases involving small children. When we walked to the pre-op area and spied the crying toddler, I felt nervous. While we interviewed the girl's parents, the feeling grew worse. I looked over at Dr. C. His lips were dry and he could barely mumble. The parents sensed our anxiety, and the mother asked Dr. C if he was comfortable with anesthetizing children. "Yes . . . I mean, of course, I've done a number of them," he replied in an embarrassed voice. It's a line that doctors sometimes use to deflect attention away from their inexperience, since technically speaking they aren't lying—their "number" is simply zero.

We left to go set up the operating room. I looked for the pediatric breathing circuit, which is smaller than the adult-sized version, but couldn't find it. Dr. C became frantic. "You can't do a pediatric case without a pediatric circuit!" he roared. In fact, you can, I found out later. But doctors out of their element often fuss about technology. They feel compelled to imitate the expert at all points lest they stray into utter darkness by deviating for an instant.

We brought the little girl into the operating room. Dr. C gave her an intramuscular injection of Atropine, a drug that increases heart rate. The drug is useful in children because their circulatory system is so rate dependent. I asked Dr. C whether the drug was necessary in this particular case. Dr. C said nothing. I asked again. I really wanted to learn. Finally, he barked, "Shut up, Dworkin! This is what pediatric anesthesiologists do. OK? They give Atropine." I fell silent.

Dr. C was acting silly, but I blame the system for his silliness. Dr. C had put his faith in technical expertise because professional medicine equates expertise with good doctoring. It is why Dr. C had subspecialized in neuroanesthesia—to become a technical expert. Professional medicine tells doctors to master a small bit of terrain to the exclusion of everything else, and that by doing so they will reach the heights of doctoring, in both prestige and salary. Yet all this does is turn a doctor into a monkey who performs a special trick. Dr. C's problem was that he had trained for a different trick. When the system pushed Dr. C onto the wrong stage, the monkey became an ass, which is a very different thing.

I put the mask over the child's face and slowly rotated the dial on the anesthesia canister. The child screamed. When she finally lost consciousness and entered the second stage of anesthesia, known as the "excitement" phase, her eyes diverged and she began to cough. To make matters worse her tongue fell back and obstructed her airway. I started to place an oral airway inside her mouth to lift the tongue off the back of her throat, but Dr. C stayed my hand. "Don't! You'll cause laryngospasm!" he shouted excitedly. (In laryngospasm, a complication of stage-two anesthesia, the patient's irritated vocal cords clamp together spasmodically, preventing air from passing through into the lungs.) What Dr. C said was true—in adults. Small children respond differently to an oral airway, a pediatric anesthesiologist had once told me. "Remember that," she had said to drive the point home, as one day I might find myself in the very trouble I was in now. I explained this to Dr. C, who relented. The oral airway worked like a charm.

When the child was deep enough, Dr. C inserted an intravenous in her arm. I tried to intubate her but failed. Dr. C also tried and failed. He then tried to breathe for the child with a bag and mask, but secretions elicited during the intubation attempts, combined with a return to stage-two anesthesia, caused the child to go into laryngospasm. Her airway was now completely obstructed. The child's heart rate dropped into the fifties. Dr. C's eyes stared into space with a newfound intensity. The surgeon scented danger.

"Do something!" the surgeon shouted.

Dr. C hesitated. "Perhaps . . . perhaps . . . we can try some Atropine?" he ventured meekly.

"She doesn't need Atropine! She needs oxygen!" blared the surgeon. He was correct. Low oxygen levels cause a child's heart rate to drop.

I hurriedly injected succinylcholine, a rapid-acting muscle relaxant, into the intravenous to relax the girl's vocal cords. Within thirty seconds Dr. C was able to ventilate her. The oxygen bolus quickly returned her heart rate to normal.

Dr. C again tried to intubate the child. This time he was successful. He breathed a sigh of relief as he listened with his stethoscope to confirm that the tube was in the right place. Then he looked at me with smiling eyes. He seemed to feel a certain pleasure knowing that a big part of this important business was already over. He even grew proud enough to teach me a few pointers about pediatric anesthesia.

When the surgeon finished the repair everyone was in good spirits. Nothing else, it seemed, could go wrong. But catastrophes do occur at the end of a case precisely because it is a time when doctors and nurses relax and let their guards down. They think of other things and their powers of concentration wane. After the surgeon wrapped the little leg in gauze I removed the child's breathing tube. Instead of breathing normally, as she had when the tube was in place, she held her breath. Maybe she was breathing but her breaths were too small to be detected, Dr. C mused aloud with a sad, almost wistful longing in his voice. He had been so happy; things had been going so well; it seemed almost unfair to him that with the case now over the gods would visit another complication on him. The temptation to ignore things at the end of a case is great—and Dr. C wanted to ignore them. But the child was definitely not breathing.

Life tensed. I nervously repositioned the little head. Fortunately, a simple chin lift made all the difference, and the child began to breathe normally again. The operating room staff breathed a sigh of relief. But the jolt had robbed Dr. C of his celebratory mood.

After the case I went back to my small on-call room, removed my shoes, and flung myself down on the narrow, springy bed. The air in the room was dry and stale; the stench of someone's lunch from earlier in the day rose from the trashcan by the brown desk. From outside the hallway the fluorescent bulb's vibrating hum sounded incessantly.

On-call rooms vary little across hospitals. Next to the bed stood a brass desk lamp with a busted shade. Years of doctors waking up disoriented in the middle of the night, reaching for the switch in the dark, and knocking the lamp over had left the shade looking like a face smashed up in a fight. By the lamp lay a phone. A brown chair claimed a corner. There was no other furniture.

I lay still on my back to avoid crumpling my facemask or losing my wallet out of my scrub shirt pocket. I wanted to sleep. When fatigue is the result of physical effort, sleep is easy, but if fatigue comes from mental effort, such as giving anesthesia, sleep is withheld despite being urgently needed. I tried to believe in my ability to sleep. I tried to imagine myself at home, spotlessly clean from a shower, in my own bed and rejoicing in my own linens. But for the next twenty minutes I stared at the red digits beaming out from the clock on the desk. It seemed to me I was the only person in the world at that moment not sleeping. I shifted my gaze toward the faint glimmer of fluorescent light peering through the bottom of the door. I began to feel the intense, clinging darkness in the room. Combined with the stale air, it felt like I had been thrown into a hole and earth was being shoveled on top of me. A heavy lump of dirt fell on my body, then another, then a third. . . .

I anxiously flicked a switch near my head, causing the overhead light to flame across the room. The first thing I saw was a large color photograph of the Vermont countryside hanging on the wall, put there to give the night call doctor a chance to wander in another, more fantastic world. Gazing at the picture I found myself drawn into the beautiful scene. I felt like the person who is suddenly infatuated with some region of the world he has never seen, but about which he is determined to learn everything— through books, through photographs. A small cabin sat in the middle of the picture. Smoke rose out of its chimney. *Perhaps a doctor lives there*, I thought. After all, serious people who do important work often go into retirement from time to time. They have country houses, mountain cabins, and cottages by the sea where they throw off all responsibility. Solitude liberates them from the actual world and lets them enter into the world of the imagination, where mundane matters recede and wider thoughts take their place. Then I looked around me, saw the busted lampshade and overflowing trashcan, and the spell was broken. In a doctor's call room solitude degrades.

I stared at my stethoscope lying on the desk, the technological symbol of doctoring, and wondered about its meaning. Is a doctor a serious person? Or is a doctor just a technician? Was I playing a great role or a small role in life? A French philosopher once said that all those who live by their work, manual or intellectual, are proletarians; all those who live by their speech he called bourgeois. Lawyers and politicians are bourgeois in that they earn their living by persuading others to pay them. Mechanics and bricklayers, by contrast, do not need to persuade—the excellence of their work is sufficient to sell it; technical knowledge replaces amiability and a slippery tongue as the source of success. But if the doctor-technician is a proletarian, he does not need nice manners. He can be rough and coarse in speech; he can dress like a tradesman, in uniform; he has no constituents, no audience—all he needs is the power to endure and work his machine. A bourgeois needs a pretty office; a proletarian can live amid trash in a call room.

So what if I were a manual laborer? Manual labor, whether it is simple or complicated, can be done well or done badly. There are clever and stupid ways of digging a hole, just as there are careful and neglectful ways of putting a person to sleep. A hole digger may do mediocre or excellent work; it depends upon his technique, his care of the shovel, his understanding of the soil, and the attention he gives to the weather. If he tries to make his work a little better than is required of him, he becomes an artist and is rewarded with more self-respect and personal enjoyment.

But unlike the manual laborer, the doctor-technician cannot really improve on his work. An anesthesiologist, for example, is expected to put a patient to sleep and wake the patient up, safely. He can do worse—catastrophically worse—but no better. A healthy, living patient is expected of him each time. Theoretically, an anesthesiologist should be as proud of his success in making his operating room into a perfect little world as a hole digger of his in digging a hole, or a diplomat of his in organizing a country's affairs. But the anesthesiologist has no real room to improve or embellish, and no reason to do any more than is necessary. The hole-digger hand paints a beautiful flower on the walls of his hole, without any relation to technique, and becomes a free artist, compared to the anesthesiologist, who never really passes beyond the boundary of technique, and never has any reason to do so.

The doctor-technician is a proletarian and a manual laborer who cannot even aspire to art, I concluded. Was this to be my calling in life? I rolled over onto my side and groaned.

I looked again at the Vermont picture. At the margin a man and woman held hands and looked into each other's eyes while standing in a field. I imagined them speaking to each other, their voices quiet, offering up declarations of love. Through the haze of my mind I pictured the glitter in the woman's questing eyes as she spoke, and the man's half-closed eyes that gleamed when he listened. I tried to imagine their interior lives. It was an odd feeling—to be using my imagination in the hospital, that is. I realized I hadn't been compelled to do so for most of my time in medicine. Every day on the wards I would memorize, reason, calculate, and estimate. I would think with my hands and manipulate objects that had weight and resistance. I would think with words and manipulate sounds and symbols to communicate a point or to prompt another person to act.

But none of this is the same as using one's imagination, where one leaves the actual world and ruminates and meditates. This may surprise, as professional medicine calls the practice of medicine an art, and art demands imagination.

Herein lies professional medicine's great mistake. Medicine *is* an art. But professional medicine confuses artistry with craftsmanship and emphasizes the latter, while only the former requires a person to be able to imagine another person's interior life.

The work of the artist is at once like and unlike that of the craftsman. Both must possess a technical expertise that can be acquired only by careful study, practice, and experience. Both the artist and the craftsman must achieve a precision of touch that enables him or her to perform a task with rapidity and complete success. During my residency, for example, I would often marvel at how fast some heart surgeons could sew in a coronary artery bypass graft. They could do so within minutes because they had been doing this all their lives. But the acquisition of technical expertise, which is essential to the craftsman (and to the monkey), is only a part of the work of the artist. The artist must pour something of himself, of his experiences, into his labor. A composer, for example, knows the form of the symphony, but he also pours his soul into the symphony. In other words, the artist, unlike the craftsman, must have lived.

So must the doctor. The doctor's life includes the actual technical part, but it also includes an imaginative part that teaches him what people are like, as well as a meditative part in which he chews the cud of his past life in order to transform his knowledge of people into medical decisions. This makes living, reading, and conversation as necessary for the doctor as learning technology.

I flicked off the light switch and lay back down on my side. I gave myself the freedom to imagine the girl in the picture. I wondered what she was like. For a young heterosexual male doctor alone in an on-call room, nothing is more desired in the middle of the night than a woman to share his bed, to caress him, to rub his leg with the soles of her feet. I began to imagine a pretty woman I had known in college, her way of fixing her hair, her smile. I felt a sudden yearning, and the effect of her memory on my body startled me. All these thoughts bombarding my consciousness exhausted me. But now, rather than welcome sleep, I fought it, eager to pore over old memories. Eventually, losing the struggle, I dozed off, my wakeful dreaming merging into semi-conscious hallucinations. I imagined a pretty woman alone, standing amid Vermont's blindingly brilliant autumn foliage, surrounded by the murmurs of the forest, the white, wind-driven clouds overhead. She was wearing a simple cotton dress, her hair was long and flowing, strands pulled back on each side in wings and held together by brown barrettes. My heart trembled with gladness; I wanted to run to her, but my strength failed me, or something restrained me, and the most I could do was move in little spurts. Her image began to fade, and I wondered how I was going to live in this forest alone. An invincible terror took possession of me. I strained harder; I prayed to whoever was holding me for mercy, groaning and cursing.

Then my beeper stuttered insistently and angrily.

The real world was calling. Time to get up. . . .

I called the number on the screen. It was the emergency room. The doctor on the other end of the line said that a patient was having difficulty breathing and might need to be intubated.

I went to evaluate her. The woman was in her twenties, thin, and wearing a party dress. She had asked her friend to take her home because she was feeling feverish and her throat hurt. While in the car she grew short of breath, so her friend made a quick detour to the hospital. When I met her she was sitting bolt upright in a tripod position, her head leaning forward and her arms extended in front of her, her fists bracing against the gurney. All her energy was focused on getting air into her lungs; even her saliva was ignored, as she let it drool down the sides of her mouth. Her eyes were unmoved, unseeing, and inexpressive. When I introduced myself a look of helpless bewilderment passed over her face in a sort of anxious spasm, making her sentient for an instant, only to return again to that look of dumb amazement.

Her symptoms suggested acute epiglottitis, where the inflamed organ sitting above the windpipe blocks air from passing into the lungs. This confused me, as I thought epiglottitis was a disease of children. Nevertheless, an X-ray of her neck confirmed the diagnosis. The situation was urgent. The woman needed to have an artificial airway established in the operating room before the inflamed tissue closed off her windpipe altogether.

When I went upstairs and told Dr. C about the case, he turned pale and looked at his watch. It was five o'clock in the morning. Perhaps the case might be delayed until seven, when the regular day would start and more staff would be around, he wondered out loud. I rolled my eyes. Then he pulled himself together and announced the plan:

Acute epiglottitis is usually a pediatric problem, he noted. Therefore we would apply the strategy that pediatric anesthesiologists use in such cases. We would breathe the woman down with anesthetic gas; when she was deep enough, we would intubate her. To be safe, we would have an ENT surgeon around, ready to open a hole in her neck in case the airway closed off altogether before the tube could be inserted.

A modest plan, but in retrospect it was not realizable. Again, Dr. C's error was to copy pediatric anesthesiologists at all points and not dare to stray. Our patient exhibited stridor, meaning she made a vibrating noise with each inhalation because her airway had narrowed. Because a child's airway is already narrow it takes only slight additional narrowing to cause stridor; hence the endotracheal tube size needed in a stridorous child may be only slightly less than that needed in a healthy child. Moreover, the alternative to intubation—placing a hole in the windpipe directly through the neck, a procedure called *tracheostomy*—is fraught with post-operative complications in children. This is why pediatric anesthesiologists prefer to intubate children suffering from acute epiglottitis. Stridor in an adult, however, indicates a high degree of narrowing. The normal adult airway is fifteen to twenty millimeters in diameter, but an adult will not exhibit stridor until his or her airway is less than five millimeters in diameter—a large drop in cross-sectional area. Only a tiny breathing tube relative to normal size can pass through a stridorous adult's narrowed airway, leaving the adult with the impossible task of breathing through a thin straw. Much safer to let a surgeon carefully and methodically place a wide-bore tracheostomy in an adult's neck while the adult is still awake, especially since adults suffer fewer postoperative complications from tracheostomies than children do.

But Dr. C wasn't thinking that way. He was a pseudo-technician trying to mimic a real technician. He was a monkey on the wrong stage.

Although he had a plan, Dr. C showed signs of uneasiness. Instead of waiting calmly for the moment to strike, he did his utmost to avoid it, to put it off and to keep it at a distance from him. When the ward clerk asked him if she should send for the patient, Dr. C said he needed more time to set up the operating room. When the nurse finished sterilizing the instruments, he told her to run them through the autoclave again, to be safe. He was trying to run out the clock; he was trying to get to 7 AM. His instinct for self-preservation was strong. It is the same instinct that fills a man sentenced to death with hopes that are not destined not be fulfilled. Dr. C kept looking anxiously at his watch, as if expecting it to save him. He seemed to know that his expectations were in vain, but he waited all the same.

The patient arrived. The ENT resident arrived a minute later. He was a good-looking young man with that look of self-satisfaction and conceit that senior residents are often more likely to exhibit than to deserve. He stood near the operating room table with a bored air. When Dr. C asked him whether he was ready to place a tracheostomy quickly, he replied, "Of course. No problem." I detected something of the patronizing attitude of the expert standing above the rest of humanity in the tone of his reply, which was jarring, since he was a resident, as was I, but Dr. C either failed to notice it or simply overlooked it.

It was Dr. C's second mistake—again, the mistake of the craftsman, not the artist. Dr. C was obsessed with technique and ignorant of what life experience should have been screaming to him about this young man: how this young man had yet to lose the freewheeling habits of his student days; how he had retained the urge to brag, to feign omniscience, and to conceal with casual aloofness any personal doubts about his abilities; how this young man proudly felt he was not like other young men. I recognized the personality from my college years: mental laziness combined with a rapscallion's hope that "something always turns up, not to worry." The young man could not be taken at his word! But Dr. C failed to take his measure and wrongly put his trust in him.

We put the woman at a forty-five degree angle on the operating room table. She made a long and melancholy cry with each inspiration. The sound seemed to arise from the very depths of her being. As the nurse prepped the neck, the woman fixed her eyes on the operating room light overhead, as if thinking here was the center, the focus around which the world gravitated. She was oblivious to the activities going on around her. She seemed to know only that something strong and bright, but less bright than sunny warmth, swept her face, and that she needed more air.

I placed the mask on her face and turned up the gas. Gradually, the anesthetic tugged at her consciousness, inducing forgetfulness, lassitude.

Then came darkness, deep and impenetrable, weighing heavily on her brain. I thought she would be resigned to the darkness, to be almost grateful for it. But she was not resigned. There was some instinct in her that desperately craved freedom from the blackness. Although unconscious, she snapped her head from side to side. She reached for the mask with an arm I had forgotten to tie down. She defiantly withheld her breath.

Finally, she settled down. Then I looked inside her mouth with my laryngoscope. I saw only red, angry-looking tissue. I could not find the hole where I needed to insert my tube. I asked Dr. C to bang on the woman's chest to send a small air bubble out of her windpipe, to act as a beacon. I confidently placed my tube at what I thought was the exit point. But my monitors quickly told me that my tube had gone into the esophagus and not the trachea. Dr. C furiously pushed me aside. His eyes darted back and forth, disturbed and restless. He tried to intubate the patient but failed. He tried a second time and failed again. Three attempts at intubation had irritated the woman's already inflamed epiglottis, further narrowing the hole she had to breathe through. Nevertheless, air still squeaked through.

This is when the catastrophe occurred—a catastrophe that followed directly from Dr. C's misunderstanding of what a doctor is. Professional medicine says a doctor is a craftsman, a technical expert. Therefore, Dr. C assumed, a good doctor must be a good craftsman who can perform a craftsman's technical tasks. It would be a failure of doctoring not to do so, he believed. It was on such thinking that one more attempt at intubation hinged. Dr. C could have ordered the ENT resident to start work on a tracheostomy now, while the woman was still breathing. That way the resident could have taken his time. But Dr. C was tempted to try one more time to intubate, to prove to the whole world he was a doctor.

I have watched this mind-set operate in other venues. Anesthesiologists, for example, are keenly conscious of who is superior in the art of spinal and epidural anesthesia. When an anesthesiologist successfully places a spinal needle in a patient after another anesthesiologist has failed, the failed anesthesiologist feels like a man unable to consummate his marriage. He feels impotent, he can't penetrate, he can't get the thing in, and another man must do it for him. He endures a serious challenge to his manhood, and although he appreciates the other anesthesiologist's help, he also hates him for succeeding.

This mind-set is especially dangerous when it involves intubations. The egos of some anesthesiologists are tied up with being technical wizards. Because they associate being a doctor with performing a procedure, they will jam a breathing tube inside a patient's airway again and again, determined to get the tube in, causing so much throat swelling that the patient suffocates. I am familiar with several such patient deaths around the country.

It was on this mind-set that our patient's life hinged. Already shamed by his lack of pediatric anesthesia expertise, Dr. C was determined to salvage his reputation by accomplishing a more difficult trick: intubating a patient with acute epiglottitis. "There was a man!" he imagined the crowd would roar. In fact, there was a monkey. He placed the breathing tube in the woman's throat a fourth time. When the monitors proved again that the tube was in the wrong place, he quickly removed it and put the mask over the woman's face to let her breathe oxygen and anesthetic gas, but now she was completely obstructed. Instead of her chest rising when she tried to breathe, it sank. Within seconds her color grew dusky.

All of us knew instinctively that death was close. Dr. C barked at the ENT resident, "Do the trach!"

The resident's face grew white as a sheet. "Okay, but you know, I actually haven't done this before . . ." he pleaded.

Slowly, as if trying to remember the illustrations in a textbook, the resident cut the delicate throat with a scalpel. The more layers he penetrated, the more blood flowed from the small wound and poured over the sides onto the mottled neck. The patient's anatomy was deranged, he declared, to justify his slow pace. After a minute, no real progress had been made. The resident began to poke aimlessly in search of hard cartilaginous rings. The patient was turning blue. Her heart rate dropped into the forties.

Drops of sweat chilled my back. I looked at Dr. C. His nervous eyes had a hint of madness in them as he gazed back at me. "Perhaps we can give her some Atropine?" he panted with agitation. She didn't need Atropine; she needed oxygen. But Dr. C injected the drug through the woman's intravenous all the same.

The ENT resident dug deeper into the mashed blue-blood tissues, the blood clots themselves impersonating vital structures, with light barely able to penetrate the dark incision. A drop of brow sweat fell into his right eye. He blinked furiously to regain his vision. In the background we

heard the patient's heart rate rise on the EKG monitor. False hope: the
Atropine Dr. C had given had artificially boosted the rate, although the
underlying cause—lack of air—remained uncorrected. Irrational, deluding himself into thinking he had time when he actually had none, the ENT
resident began poking about the neck with less urgency and with a clarity
of mind that was useful but undeserved.

Things were going nowhere. I grabbed an intravenous catheter and
went to the side opposite of where the resident was working. My plan was
to pierce the small cricothyroid membrane that covers the windpipe low
in the neck, and to hook the catheter up to a high-pressure jet ventilator.
That way I could force air into the lungs, although how air would then
escape the lungs I wasn't quite sure. I was counting on the resident
carving a hole in the trachea by that time. My needle hovered over the
patient's neck below the site where the resident was working.

Suddenly a man in street clothes darted into the room. He shoved the
resident aside, grabbed a knife, and started cutting on the woman's neck.
It was the ENT attending who had been paged to come in from home.
When he had heard what was happening he skipped changing into scrubs.
Probably he had a more sober and accurate view of the ENT resident's
character than Dr. C did, adding to his sense of urgency. Within twenty
seconds the windpipe rose out of the wound. The surgeon cut horizontally
between two rings. He snatched a hook to spread the incision apart and
then inserted a tracheostomy tube into the hole. I connected the tube to
the anesthesia circuit and forced pure oxygen into the patient's lungs.
Everyone fell back for a few moments and gazed at the patient's face,
once blue, now reassuringly pale white—a mask that perhaps concealed
some deeper damage within.

We brought the patient to the recovery room. She had yet to regain
consciousness. Dr. C looked around skittishly to see if any eyes accused
him.

I stood staring at the woman, girlishly pretty even in her critical state.
She still wore her party dress. The arm that had reached up for the mask
during the anesthetic induction lay on the gurney, its hand clenched tight.
In all the swirling activity we had missed it, and I peeled back the fingers

to reveal a tiny locket with a young man's picture in it. Evidently she had clutched the locket before arriving in the emergency room.

"Who—who were you dreaming of in your hour of doom? Your boyfriend? Your brother?" I asked myself, my heart fluttering with uneasy curiosity.

I looked at her again. Life was seething, surging, pulsating inside her. Her organs were healthy and fresh. Her brain was sunk in wearisome sleep, waiting, hoping to be awakened, but the many minutes without oxygen might prevent that from happening. Nausea welled up inside me. I closed the woman's hand around the locket, deciding it was right for the locket and the woman not to be separated.

We were in the realm of the indefinite, without certainty. I was uncomfortable—and yet discomfort captures the essence of what had gone wrong. When doctors become craftsmen, they narrow down their minds to materially determined magnitudes and formulas. To be certain about what they do know, they shrink down what they have to know. But a doctor-craftsman is dangerous, as the craftsman, unlike the monkey, has an ego that needs to be stroked; the craftsman may persist in an activity long after the monkey has abandoned it. When the craftsman's work depends on knowing people, the situation grows especially dire, as people exemplify the indefinite more than anything else. The craftsman is not an artist; he or she has little understanding of other people's lives; he or she has much perfect knowledge but little imperfect knowledge; he or she is uncomfortable with the indefinite. Doctors are sometimes called "craftsmen who love humanity," but what good comes from loving humanity without knowing people? Far safer for a doctor to despise humanity but know well the people around him.

Professional medicine largely ignores the problem of subspecialists suddenly thrust onto the general stage. Doctors confess their concerns to each other privately but rarely publicly. Most medical boards today issue time-limited certifications, requiring doctors to stay abreast of their fields and keep a hand in general practice, thereby giving lip service to the problem while covering themselves at the same time. The method is useless.

I am a living example. Before anesthesiology trainees start their residencies they take the board certification exam, which they must pass three years later to become board-certified. The test at this stage is only practice; they aren't expected to pass. But I did pass. People called it a fluke. But I had read all the anesthesia textbooks the year before. It was no fluke. Nevertheless, the notion that I was a fully functioning anesthesiologist at this juncture was ridiculous. I had book knowledge but no experience in giving anesthesia. And I certainly didn't understand people. I was unsafe. In the same way, Dr. C had book knowledge about pediatric anesthesia but no experience in giving it. And he didn't know people. He could have passed a pediatric anesthesia certification test, but it would have meant nothing.

Sometimes subspecialization in medicine goes so far that instead of fearing what they no longer know, doctors cease to know that they no longer know. They grow so removed from general medicine that they no longer take other fields seriously. This also causes catastrophes. I am familiar with several cases in outpatient surgery centers where gastroenterologists or plastic surgeons supervised nurse anesthetists, having assumed the role of anesthesiologist (which they are legally allowed to do, since they are MDs), resulting in a patient death. They watch the nurse anesthetists perform their technical tasks; the whole thing looks so easy, and pushing the anesthesiologist out of the picture saves money, so, these physicians think to themselves, why not take over the supervisory role? Then a catastrophe occurs. In one case, a patient's surgery was performed in the prone position under deep sedation, which most anesthesiologists would have avoided because of the patient's large size. In another case the drug succinylcholine was not available to treat a patient's laryngospasm when her vocal cords were touched under anesthesia, causing her to suffocate. Again, the gastroenterologist was supervising the nurse anesthetist; no anesthesiologist was immediately present. Very few anesthesiologists would have performed such a case without having succinylcholine in the room. But in this case it was the gastroenterologist's call.

Fortunately, my patient finally woke up in the recovery room, her mind intact. Catastrophe had been averted. At 8 AM we all went home.

Dr. C learned nothing from the experience, except to be wilier in the future when ducking hard cases. His most trusted method came to be "discovering" a small thyroid nodule in a patient that he didn't want to put to sleep, and then demanding a full workup, thereby punting the case to another doctor at a future date. Another method of his was to hide the patient's chart before surgery to run out the clock. The nurse would waste time looking for the chart; the patient could not be brought into the operating room without it; with every minute of delay, Dr. C was that much closer to being relieved by another doctor.

I went the other way. I learned to keep a familiarity with general anesthesia practice and never to allow myself to become an exclusive sub-subspecialist. A doctor is *not* a craftsman, and a good doctor is more than just a good craftsman.

4

WHEN NO ONE IS IN COMMAND

After I finished my training, I spent time at a hospital on the East Coast. It was a period of great turmoil in doctor-nurse relations. Some nurses viewed the age-old doctors' right to boss them around and deny them patient care responsibilities as an unfair expression of doctors' might. Some doctors, in turn, viewed nurses as uppity and rebellious, and scheming to put themselves on a par with physicians. Doctors and nurses, once allies, increasingly became rivals and suspicious of one another.

During my fourth week on the job I worked with a nurse anesthetist—a noisy person, bitter and insolent. She was fielding a question from our patient as I approached from behind.

"What exactly is the difference between a nurse anesthetist and an anesthesiologist?" the patient asked innocently.

"Oh, about $300,000 a year," the nurse anesthetist replied scornfully.

I raised an eyebrow but said nothing. Later, during the case, I asked the nurse to measure the patient's blood sugar. When I returned thirty minutes later the test had not been done. I told her I was angry. Without even bothering to look at me, she replied, "Oh, go suck an egg."

I was annoyed but said nothing. I went back to the lounge and sat for a while, nursing my grievance. When a more senior doctor walked in I explained to him what had happened. He wisely told me to let the matter drop. I said I wanted to talk to the head of nursing about it. He grew pale and said that would be dangerous. Nurse X, the head of nursing, he explained, was a real bruiser.

I had heard about Nurse X. She reportedly sat in a large office at a large desk with two framed diplomas hanging on the wall behind her, one her BSN, the other her MSN.[1] She behaved like a typical self-important bureaucrat, assigning committee work to subordinates and demanding weekly written reports, even though no such committees or reports had ever been needed at the hospital. Seared with an unshakeable hatred for the old system that had doctors on top and nurses on the bottom, she spoke often about the glorious future of nursing as if she were lecturing from a rostrum. Nurses and doctors were converging on a common professional role, she argued. On the wards she wore a long white lab coat, like a doctor. For medical people, a person in a different coat seems like a different person, and so her attire was significant.

She carried out her revolution through signed memoranda. In those early days of change, nurses wielded power not by taking charge of patients but by writing policy. Some policies involved manpower and resource allocation, affecting everyone in the hospital, including doctors. A surgeon, for example, couldn't operate unless the operating room was open and a nurse was available. This depended on policy. Other policies governed how people behaved. Here, Nurse X wielded less power, since she couldn't actually command a doctor to do anything. Even in the operating room she might strongly encourage a doctor to put up his mask, but if he refused, she could do little about it, while if an orderly or technician refused, he could be immediately fired. Nurse X put out several memoranda a week covering the entire range of hospital policy, with every document signed with her name, followed by the appellation, "BSN, MSN." Employees coughed and fidgeted when reading her memos, sometimes laughing nervously among each other, referring to Nurse X as simply "BSN, MSN," and with an uneasy feeling that they might have something to fear from this person in the future. Fear as such had not yet manifested itself, except for those assigned to one of Nurse X's committees, but it was somewhere on the way, like a storm cloud billowing in from the distant horizon. Doctors also sensed trouble and avoided her as much as possible.

I decided to forget the nurse anesthetist's insult. The vast majority of nurse anesthetists I had worked with were solid professionals, and not like this nurse, so why not? However, two days later I found myself working with her again. Our patient was an elderly woman going for a D and C,[2] and possible laparoscopy, depending on what the surgeon found during the first procedure. The patient was anemic (the gynecologist thought from postmenopausal bleeding); she also had a pacemaker, diabetes, and a history of congestive heart failure. The nurse anesthetist was about to bring the patient into the operating room when I told her to hold off, as I wanted to make a few phone calls to check out the patient's pacemaker. The nurse anesthetist rolled her eyes and impatiently asked, "What for? It's working."

"If the gynecologist uses the electrocautery, we may have to put a magnet on the pacemaker," I replied.

"So . . . we'll have a magnet ready," the nurse anesthetist declared mockingly. "Besides, the gynecologist won't be using cautery during the D and C. Let's just go in."

I explained my concerns. First, I didn't know how old the pacemaker battery was. Second, if we put a magnet on the pacemaker so that it worked with the electrocautery, it would convert the pacemaker to a fixed rate. Typically that's not a problem, but if the pacemaker were a sequential model, causing the patient's atrium to beat first and then her ventricle, the fixed rate mode would lack the atrium component, which some heart failure patients need to maintain blood pressure. I couldn't tell the pacemaker type from the EKG strip, as the patient's heart was still beating on its own. Third, the patient's pacemaker might be one of those that must be reprogrammed after a magnet has been applied. I needed to find these things out.

The nurse anesthetist remained unconvinced. "But we're not even going to need the magnet," she pleaded. I held my ground. The nurse replied, "Listen, Ron, you're fresh out of the university. I've been doing this for twenty years. I've never even used a magnet."

The nurse's counterattack was cleverly two-pronged. First, she had called me "Ron" and not "Dr. Dworkin." As a resident I had allowed several nurses to address me in this way, thinking that the casual, informal, we're-all-just-friends mode was best for working relations. I realized my error during a near catastrophe when I had to order a nurse to send for blood. The nurse, lulled into believing we were professional equals, and thinking it rude for friends to order each other around, refused to obey me because she thought the blood transfusion unnecessary. Only by growing officious and harsh, and threatening her with a charge of insubordination, did I make her comply, although my harshness neutralized her contempt and turned it into hatred. A doctor must inspire respect and sometimes even a little fear among subordinates to get them to respond quickly during a crisis. Subordinates must know there are consequences to not following orders. This means preventing subordinates from taking liberties even privately, such as using a doctor's first name. True, it is hard for doctors to keep the right balance between the reserve and solemnity necessary to their positions and the affability required of them in working with subordinates, especially in a democratic society. But that just shows how a doctor must be more than a craftsman. He or she must also exercise tact.

By using my first name, the nurse anesthetist had tried to equalize our relations so that I might be more easily swayed. Citing her greater experience was another strategy. To her mind, twenty years of experience canceled out my book smarts and extended educational experience, making for a rough parity between us. In fact, this judgment is sometimes reasonable. The doctor, no matter what stage he or she is at, must have the tact, openness, and confidence to decide.

In this case, I refused to budge. The nurse anesthetist stormed off. In the distance I saw her huddle with the three other nurses. A howl of scorn arose from the small assembly. I knew they were talking about me.

I began to feel uneasy. After all, I was new at the hospital. And it was four against one. When they walked toward me I felt that my nurse anesthetist had unleashed an angry mob.

They crowded around me. One nurse declared, "This is silly. We could be waiting an hour for that rep to call." A second nurse demanded, "What makes you think you can just shut everything down?" The other two nurses nodded their heads in agreement.

I knew why the nurses were pushing me. Just as some doctors are impatient and want to go home, so are some nurses. The case was scheduled to start at 3 PM. The nurses ended their shifts at 4 PM. If the case start was delayed and the anesthetic induction and surgical prep were still going on at 4 PM, the nurses would have to stay longer to finish those activities before a new team could relieve them. They didn't want to stay. They wanted to leave exactly at 4 PM.

The assembly exerted a strange mental force on me. It started to hypnotize me, upset my equilibrium; there was no obvious reason for me to submit to it, and yet I could only keep from submitting to it by offering tremendous inward resistance. A doctor fighting another doctor is a low-intensity battle compared to a doctor fighting a nurse. A doctor may incur the wrath of another doctor, but he or she will see that other doctor only sporadically, making any workplace tension intermittent. In addition, the fight remains at the level of two combatants. But a doctor and a nurse see each other every day. When they fight, the resulting tension becomes constant and unremitting. Word of the fight soon gets around, and sometimes other nurses join the battle to defend their colleague. Their collective derision can transform the doctor's life into a living hell—a hell perpetrated in countless ways, often small and insidious, and turning the doctor into a paranoid nervous wreck. At every turn he thinks the nurses are out to get him. A nurse delays his case—they're after me (even if the nurse didn't do it intentionally). A nurse fails to carry out his order—they're after me (even if the nurse forgot the order). A nurse pretends not to hear him—they're after me (even if the nurse really didn't hear the doctor). The doctor grows so unsettled that he or she can barely make it through the day.

I kept up a bold front. I calmly told the nurses that we had to wait until we gathered all the necessary information. But I also knew well enough how many times before I had yielded in like circumstances, and experience indicated that the future would resemble the past.

The nurses badgered me until my innate predisposition to hedge led me to say that we would wait ten more minutes, and that if we hadn't heard back from either the patient's cardiologist or the pacemaker company rep by then, they could bring the patient into the operating room.

After ten minutes there was still no call. The nurses started to bring the patient into the room, but my courage had returned. I said no. The exchange grew more heated. "But you said—" declared a broken-hearted nurse, in a tone of reproach. "I'm sorry, but that's how it has to be," I replied. She kept pushing. In the end I snapped at her and called her a "silly goose." The nurse fell silent, went to make a phone call, and then sat down to wait.

Within three minutes, BSN, MSN was down in the holding area, standing directly in front of me and looking very angry. She was a large and imposing person, wearing a long white lab coat.

"Young man, did you call one of my nurses a 'goose'?" she blared.

My little assembly of nurses gathered round. Feelings of detestation and horror mingled with satisfaction. This was what was wanted, it seemed. It felt as though they wanted to make me feel like a boor, rather than the knowledgeable professional I was. If I were a respected doctor, they would have to contend with me. But I had used the hated g-word. The role of archfiend in this grim drama now belonged to me. And if BSN, MSN could produce in such a spectacular manner evidence of boorishness in me, some of which didn't even need proving (given what I had said), then clearly it followed that this assembly of nurses should reject all my recommendations in regard to the patient, who should be brought into the operating room forthwith.

There was a stir of anxiety. The assembly sensed this was the big moment: this was the moment when I would either seize the leading role or be put in my place for good.

Still smarting over my nurse having told me a few days before to go suck an egg, I refused to cave.

"Did I call the nurse a goose? I'm not sure. Maybe I just said she was something like a goose," I replied with heavy sarcasm.

"Now you listen here—" BSN, MSN said before stopping herself and proceeding in a more pedantic tone of voice. "Now listen, young man, our job is to take care of patients. We're a team. Do you understand? We all want what's best for the patient. To work as a team we must treat each other with respect."

I told the chief nurse that I understood her concerns, but I also explained my concerns regarding the pacemaker and the pushback I'd been getting from her nurses.

BSN, MSN winked at the nurses, feeling herself to be on firmer footing. "Waiting so long for this rep to call does seem unreasonable. I think we should at least start the case," she declared with confidence. It was now five against one.

"Well, I think differently. And I'm the doctor, so I'm in charge," I replied firmly.

"In charge of me?" she asked, her suspicions flaming up again.

"In this situation I am," I said.

BSN, MSN stood still for a few moments in silence. "I'm not subordinate to you, young man," she harshly interjected.

"Then who are you subordinate to?" I asked.

"I am subordinate to the hospital president and to the board. You're in a department. I run a department. We're equal. Don't forget that," she answered angrily.

A phone call from the pacemaker company representative interrupted the standoff. The rep said the patient's pacemaker was a standard one, not a sequential one. It did not have to be reprogrammed after magnet placement. The battery was fresh. The nurses felt vindicated. My concerns had been for nothing, although we could not have known this before the phone call. But the nurses didn't see it that way. They already had a claim on me for my name-calling; now, to their minds, their judgment on medical matters had proved superior to mine.

BSN, MSN joined in the triumph, smiling even while her eyes still blazed furiously. Pointing her forefinger at the syringe in my shirt pocket, she said, "That's an unlabeled syringe, doctor. You know the rules. All syringes must be labeled." She was determined to drive the point home that we were on equal footing, that each of us could take turns ordering the other, that she was watching me carefully and was prepared for any eventuality, and that it would be unwise for me to come into conflict with her again.

The nurses brought the patient into the operating room. I started the case by myself, my nurse anesthetist having left for the day. I placed the monitors on the patient and gave her some intravenous sedation. Two operating room nurses hoisted the patient's legs into stirrups. Both were new to the case. During the hand-off the departing nurses had spent longer than usual telling the new nurses about the patient—and the reason for our delay. The four nurses had whispered quietly to each other, with one of them glancing in my direction every few seconds. Although we had entered the operating room on my terms, I knew I had not regained my old position, as if there had never been a quarrel.

The gynecologist started the D and C. When I asked one of the nurses if she could get me some warm blankets to put across the patient's chest, she promptly did so. Then she left the room to start another case across the hall. I noticed that the bag of saline connected to the patient's intravenous was almost empty. Because I had to hold the sleeping patient's chin to assist her breathing, I asked the remaining nurse to grab a fresh bag from the cabinet for me. The nurse acted as if she could neither see nor hear me. I dropped the patient's chin and got the bag myself.

I understood everything. It was the struggle between doctor and nurse—who would dominate whom? Nothing was fixed, everything was fluid and precarious, the outcome of the struggle unclear. I hoped that my decision to get the saline on my own, to be the bigger person, would appease the nurse's pride enough to smooth things over. I was wrong. Every time I asked her for help, she would project an air of disinterest or sometimes pretend not to hear; when she did pay attention, she looked at me derisively. Still, I carefully avoided pushing things into a state of open conflict, for I knew that when a doctor fights a nurse, the loss is great, while the gain is dubious.

Toward the end of the case, my semiconscious patient began to experience pain. I gave her additional intravenous sedation, but she continued to moan. I didn't want to put her completely to sleep, with a breathing tube, because her anatomy suggested she would be a difficult intubation. Putting her to sleep without a breathing tube, however, risked aspiration, because of her diabetes. It was a difficult situation, and an embarrassing one for an anesthesiologist, whose job is to eliminate pain. The prudent course, I decided, was to continue with small doses of intravenous sedation, including a drug called Versed, which causes antegrade amnesia (meaning a patient fails to consolidate into memory events going forward). Although the patient might still express pain, unconsciousness would prevent her from being aware of her pain, while Versed would keep her from remembering her pain.

Nevertheless, a moaning patient looks bad. The nurse came over and demanded that I put the patient to sleep. I tried to explain to her my thinking while simultaneously watching the monitors and injecting more drugs. She stared at me angrily. When the patient moaned again, the nurse repeated her demand, looking at me as if I were an unfeeling brute. The duel had to end. "Listen, when I want your opinion, I'll ask for it," I snapped. Then I looked away.

The gynecologist decided that uterine bleeding failed to explain the patient's anemia. There was no reason to proceed to laparoscopy. Then he performed one more pelvic exam. He suddenly exclaimed that he felt an ovarian mass in the patient for the first time. He wanted to move forward with laparoscopy after all. I was surprised—and a little suspicious. I asked him why he had suddenly detected a mass now. He replied that anesthesia often allows for a more accurate exam, as it relaxes a patient's muscles. Seemed reasonable. Still, in the back of my mind I wondered if he had just wanted an excuse to perform a laparoscopy, to gain practice, as laparoscopy was a relatively new procedure in those days. I asked him what he was hoping to find. He quietly replied, "We're just going to take a little look around."

I intubated the patient after some struggle. A technician came in to assist the surgeon. He was a young man with no more than a high school education. But he knew how to work the laparoscope better than any doctor did, as he had been trained to assist physicians on this particular surgery, and only this surgery.

The gynecologist fumbled with the laparoscopic equipment, failing to pierce the patient's abdominal wall with the needle that fills the abdominal cavity with air. He pushed too little because he feared that pushing too hard might cause the needle to puncture a major blood vessel. The technician did it for him. Once the gynecologist was inside the cavity, he moved the organs around with a long stick, causing some bleeding that short bursts of cautery stemmed. I stood ready to apply the magnet to the pacemaker, but it wasn't needed.

The gynecologist inspected the ovary that he thought had a mass. He wasn't sure if there was a mass, and he hesitated over what to do. He looked at the technician, who sensed his opinion was desired. The technician said he had seen similar situations before. Those surgeons who had dissected down further often regretted it, he noted. He recommended coming out of the abdomen and doing a more complete workup with noninvasive radiography. The technician then remained silent for a minute, and the gynecologist remained silent also. But the latter's eyes were as active as ever. He looked at the monitor that held a picture of the patient's ovary; then he allowed his eyes to settle on the surgical site. He seemed uneasy. Finally, he decided to take the technician's advice and end the surgery.

It was an odd moment. This young man had appeared unexpectedly, from out of the blue, and determined the direction of the case. He was practicing medicine. There was nothing of the doctor about him—neither the surgeon's knowledge of anatomy nor my knowledge of physiology. He was an instrument. He carried out the will of others. But because he had performed the same activity over and over again, he had gone from being an instrument to being someone able to help, advise, and decide on a particular case. If that is the definition of a doctor, then he had become a doctor.

The reader may think I am devaluing what this young man had to offer. In fact, it's just the opposite. He had added real value. As an accomplished technician, he may even represent the future of medicine. Instead, my doubts are about the doctors. If a technician with vast experience doing a particular procedure can outperform a doctor doing that procedure, then what value does the doctor add? What important contribution does the doctor make? What is distinctive about being a doctor? *Perhaps nothing*, I thought to myself as I wheeled the patient back to the recovery room.

Several days later, I drove downtown to a hotel for a medical conference on "team medicine." Attendance was compulsory for doctors, nurses, and surgical staff from the region's major hospitals, with multiple sections convening on different dates to accommodate people's schedules. The conference's purpose was to move doctors and nurses, now called "providers," toward a more democratic approach to decision making. In the future, at least in the ideal, nurses would offer advice and input, doctors would listen carefully, and the health care "team" would make decisions instead of doctors acting unilaterally.

When I walked into the large conference room, I saw faces that I recognized, looking bored or sullen. Unlike most medical meetings, where people go to enjoy themselves, to meet friends, and to be simultaneously instructed and entertained, this meeting was strictly business. On the podium sat three nurses whom I did not recognize, along with BSN, MSN. I took a seat in the back.

One of the nurses went up to the lectern and spoke generally about the meeting's purpose. She talked about the importance of helping the patient and working together to do so. She said we should treat our patients the way we would want our family members to be treated. Her words seemed unnecessary, as no one in the room—doctor, nurse, or technician— thought otherwise. The whole speech conveyed a sense of emptiness and thinness. Afterward a few people clapped.

Our first activity was designed to "break down barriers," but its real purpose was to destroy the traditional chain of command. Doctors, nurses, and orderlies were randomly divided into groups, each group containing a sampling of all three. A group's job was to grab some Legos from a large bin in the center of the room, return to home base, and build a tower with them. The group that built the highest tower at the end of five minutes would be declared the winner. Each group would have one commander, three people to run over and grab the Legos, and three people remaining at home base to build with the Legos. Who was to command and who was to obey in the tower-building process was the essential teaching point. The commander was to be chosen at random; a doctor did not automatically assume command. The commander would bark orders to subordinates, telling them, for example, that the group needed this size Lego, or two of that size, or four of another. If the commander was a nurse or an orderly, he or she would experience the thrill of ordering doctors to fetch Legos, while doctors, in turn, would learn to accept advice and direction from a lower member of the team.

The race began. A few doctors got into the spirit of things and good-naturedly ran to the Legos bin when a nurse or orderly commanded them to. But most of the doctors looked self-conscious, perceiving that the exercise's purpose was to wound their dignity and take them down a notch. Several doctors grinned on purpose to keep from sneering as they ran toward the bin. A few doctors stared blankly into space as they ran, each of them embarrassed for the other. One elderly doctor was so insulted that he remained seated, frowning fastidiously in his chair, scouring his coat sleeve for dirt, and obviously thinking it beneath him to be treated in such a manner. As a Lego builder rather than a retriever, I was able to conceal my displeasure with slow hand motions that went unnoticed.

At the end of five minutes, the group with the two doctors who had given it their all was declared the winner. Its members cheered and returned to their seats.

A second nurse went up to the lectern. She talked about a case in which a nurse had tried to tell a doctor about a patient's new symptoms, only to have the doctor ignore her. The patient died as a result. The nurse dabbed her eye with a tissue, and then she gave two more examples of patients injured when a doctor had failed to listen to a nurse. "We can do better!" she declared.

What the nurse said was true. We can do better. I know of several cases when doctors overlooked a nurse's wise counsel and the patient suffered as a result. In one case, a nurse anesthetist suggested giving a patient a drying agent before the doctor tried to perform an awake intubation. The doctor ignored the nurse; as a result, the patient had so many oral secretions that an awake intubation proved impossible. In a second case, a nurse anesthetist suspected that a patient had eaten before surgery. She suggested canceling the case, or at least placing a breathing tube to protect against aspiration. The doctor refused to listen to her; the case was done under mask anesthesia; in the end, the patient did aspirate and ended up in the intensive care unit for two weeks.

But the nurse at the conference was after something different. Her sadness, her irritation, her enthusiasm—it was all laid bare for us. Everyone in the audience knew what was going on and quietly submitted to the invisible process. They knew a new belief system, the team system, was being drummed into their heads. That new system aspired to put doctors and nurses on the same level.

Ironically, this new belief system is as flawed as the old belief system that held doctors to be omniscient and unassailable. Both belief systems substitute a lofty worldview for complicated reality; both see the practice of medicine as something that can be encompassed through a fundamental principle—an excellent idea, but one that is not accurate. Medical practice is a murky world of egos and personalities, of authority tempered by the natural give-and-take between people, and something best navigated using tact and common sense. A nurse with a fanatical belief in team medicine, like a doctor with a fanatical belief in his or her supremacy, is like the housekeeper with a fanatical belief in the possibility of a clean house. The housekeeper's mistake is not in fighting the dirt but in trying to get rid of it altogether, as though such a thing were possible. A house is necessarily a dirty place. Metaphorically speaking, so is medical practice. Too many human limitations prevent the application of ideology.

Privately, many in the audience resisted what the nurse was saying or approached the new system with a mixture of doubt and belief. Even some of the nurses resisted, wondering about the new system's viability in practice. They also resented being given high-minded lessons on how to live. But everyone feared a shake of the head or a warning finger from the nurse on the podium if they dared to express doubt. Indeed, faults that in other fields might have delegitimized the speaker—her strangely false and high-pitched moral tone, her melodramatic absurdities, and her belief in progress—gave her power. Everyone in the audience knew they would have to accept the new system if they wanted to continue their professional lives in a quiet, tranquil, and unruffled manner.

The nurse then told the story of how her own mother had mistakenly taken some medicine with bourbon, thinking it was doctor's orders. Her doctor had only been joking when suggesting she take it with alcohol. Indeed, the doctor's own nurse had warned the doctor that the patient might have taken the order seriously. But the doctor ignored the nurse. The woman ended up drunk.

The audience stared at the nurse with puzzled eyes, uncertain how they were to react. Should they laugh? Should they continue thinking serious thoughts? The audience looked at the other three nurses on stage to see how they were taking it. All of them were grinning. At once all doubts vanished. We should have known. This was a comedy turn. Soon we all echoed with obedient laughter.

The nurse at the lectern previewed a short film clip we were about to watch: a dramatic reenactment of a true story about an anesthesiologist in Britain who had trouble intubating a patient. Because the nurses and staff in the operating room had been too cowed to advise the doctor, the patient woke up brain-dead.

We watched the clip. Something in it didn't make sense. The actress playing the patient was thin and had a normal-looking airway. The drama skipped time in five-minute intervals, with the actor playing the anesthesiologist failing each time to intubate the patient, but also calmly breathing for the patient with bag and mask. Several nurse-actors attended the doctor. They remained silent and played the role of cowed subordinates, but what they were kept from saying that would have made a difference was unclear. The clip conveyed no sense of urgency.

Some doctors in the audience grew emboldened during the discussion that followed. One anesthesiologist queried, "If the patient was so thin and with normal airway anatomy, why did the anesthesiologist in real life have trouble intubating her?"

"I'm not sure what the problem was exactly," the nurse at the lectern replied. "But that's not the point. The point is—"

Another doctor cut her off. "It *is* the point," she said. "If the patient had been morbidly obese, requiring multiple intubation attempts, then maybe the anesthesiologist shouldn't have put her to sleep in the first place. But that was the anesthesiologist's decision. Nothing for nursing to say on the matter."

Sensing pushback and eager to rescue their cause, one of the other conference leaders walked up to the lectern. "I believe the patient was slightly above average weight. But for some reason the anesthesiologist had trouble intubating her," she explained.

"But why?" interjected an ENT surgeon, defiantly. "Even a patient with a difficult airway can usually be ventilated with a bag and mask, especially a thin one. Something doesn't sound right. I don't think nursing input would have made a difference in this case. Something else was going on that caused the patient to wake up brain-dead."

The two nurses stood at the lectern, hesitating. They appeared not to know how to react. Should they take the doctor seriously? Should they perceive some level of insult? Should they ignore the doctor? The situation seemed to be something outside their experience.

BSN, MSN approached the lectern with the third nurse. She looked angry, as if the doctors in the audience were saying the wrong things, appalling things. "The nurses were probably too afraid to tell the anesthesiologist that the patient's oxygen level was declining," BSN, MSN declared. "That's what happens when the team is not allowed—"

"But why would a doctor even have to be told?" I interrupted. "An anesthesiologist's ear is carefully trained to listen to the sound of the oxygen monitor. It's almost second nature to him; he practically hears it in his sleep. The one thing that anesthesiologist *would* have known is the patient's oxygen level."

BSN, MSN's eyes blazed. "Maybe he didn't! That's why a team's input is most needed in a crisis!" she loudly declared.

The room fell silent for a moment. An elderly African American orderly sat two seats from me on my left. I recognized him from my hospital. His hair was gray; he stooped somewhat; his face was a spiderweb of furrows; his demeanor deferential. The old system had not only prematurely aged him but also taught him that his opinion was both unwanted and undesirable. But at this moment, years of operating room experience seemed to stir his conscience. I heard him quietly mutter under his breath, "I disagree."

A brassy, middle-aged OB/GYN sitting in front of me was more vocal. In a sneering tone she shouted at BSN, MSN, "When anesthesia is having a problem, it's not time to talk. It's time to shut the fuck up!"

BSN, MSN looked furious. Staring fixedly and authoritatively at the audience, she declared, "Now let me tell you, people, that so far as the future is concerned, it's going to be like this. We're going to work as a team, got it? The team has rules. If you've got sense, follow them, but if you haven't, clear out."

In a stern voice, she went on about what nurses had to offer the team, both as patient caregivers and as advocates. Never in my life had I seen a more vicious caricature of nursing love. All of it resembled what nurses do, but at the same time, for some inexplicable reason, it was so unpleasant that the audience did not utter another word. On the faces of all were confusion and concern.

Two weeks later, the patient with the unexplained anemia returned to the hospital for removal of a tumor in her small intestine. Nurse A, the nurse anesthetist on the case with me, was a young man in his mid-thirties, technically adept, confident, sometimes a bit too confident, knowing what he knew without knowing what he didn't know. One might have called him naive. He had the habit of mentally brushing aside advice from his supervising physician, thinking himself quite capable of working independently. He knew this attitude irritated his supervisors, but for him, that irritation was only a sign that the advantage was *on his side*.

We decided to place an arterial line preoperatively in the holding area. This involves inserting an intravenous catheter into one of the arteries at the wrist and connecting it to a pressure monitor, yielding instantaneous blood pressure measurements. I tried placing the catheter in the patient's left radial artery—twice—but failed. Nurse A was eager to try. I gave him the green light after my second failed attempt. He quickly placed the line in the patient's right radial artery and was barely able to conceal his self-satisfaction in doing so.

But he had gotten the line in.

During the case, the patient's IV through her vein stopped working, and because no other peripheral vein was visible, we decided to place a central line to regain venous access. Nurse A asked if he could perform the procedure. I agreed. He bent the patient's wrinkled neck to the left and swept across its right surface with antiseptic. Then he broke the patient's skin with a well-aimed puncture, eliciting a sudden flash of blood. He passed a flexible wire through the needle, and then passed the long catheter over the wire toward the right side of the patient's heart. He did a nice job.

Shortly after, we checked the patient's blood sugar. It measured 230. I directed Nurse A to give the patient a small dose of insulin and then left the operating room. When I returned ten minutes later, the patient's EKG showed frequent premature beats that risked turning into a dangerous arrhythmia. When I scanned the monitor that measures the level of carbon dioxide in a patient's breath and saw the number 30 on the screen, I instinctively knew what had happened.

Insulin drives potassium levels down. So does blood alkalosis. The normal carbon dioxide level in human beings is 40. Breathing slower than normal raises carbon dioxide and makes blood more acidic, while breathing faster than normal lowers carbon dioxide and makes blood more alkalotic. Nurse A was ventilating the patient at twelve times a minute and causing a respiratory alkalosis. The patient's potassium level, already low to begin with (at 3.5), had declined from insulin, and declined further from alkalosis, causing dangerous ventricular ectopy.

I dropped the ventilator rate from twelve to six, which corrected the problem. Nurse A said nothing, but I was angry. He had been hyperventilating the patient for no obvious reason. And yet I was more to blame than he was for the trouble.

Many doctors prefer to do everything themselves, since all orders can be misunderstood. But that's not possible today. There aren't enough doctors. Instead, doctors must supervise the work of nurses and other physician extenders. They must know how to use the minds of others. For this reason they must take into account both the tradition and the custom of the workplace in which they practice. Every nurse anesthetist at my hospital, and not just Nurse A, moderately hyperventilated their patients as a matter of course. It was their custom. I had observed this, and I should have foreseen the consequences of treating my patient with insulin in this environment. It is not enough for a doctor give an order. A doctor must see to its execution and, when giving it, anticipate anything that may nullify its effectiveness. Custom has a terrible way of avenging itself when violated.

I told Nurse A to call me if there were any more problems. Then I left the room to check on another case. I wandered back an hour later. Nurse A had just turned off the anesthetic gas and was waiting for the patient to wake up. It seemed to take longer than usual. Also, the patient's blood pressure was 83/50, lower than expected during a wake-up.

"What's going on?" I asked.

"I'm not sure," replied Nurse A. "I turned off the gas and gave the drugs to reverse the muscle relaxant, but she's not waking up."

"Are you sure you gave her reversal and not something else?" the surgeon asked with an accusatory tone.

"Yeah, I'm sure," replied Nurse A, defensively.

We waited a few more minutes. The patient remained unconscious as her blood pressure continued to sag.

"For God's sake, what did you give her?" the surgeon shouted angrily at Nurse A.

"I told you. I gave the reversal," he replied, but this time with doubt in his voice. "I know it didn't cause her blood pressure to drop," he added with more self-assurance. "That started before I gave the reversal."

I jumped in. "Why didn't you call me?" I asked.

"I knew what I was doing," replied Nurse A proudly. "I checked the central line pressure. It was 10 mm. I figured the gas was depressing her heart, and that things would get better when I turned it off."

I pulled down the patient's lower eyelid. Her conjunctiva was paler, and less pink, than when we had started.

"What are you doing?" barked the surgeon.

"She looks more anemic than before," I mused.

"We didn't lose that much blood," said the surgeon, defensively.

"I'm just saying she looks more anemic," I replied.

"It's probably from the low blood pressure," insisted Nurse A.

There is something that exists in anesthesiologists beyond the realm of consciousness, some mysterious clocklike mechanism that suddenly gives a signal when trouble looms. Call it a weird prescience or instinct; whatever it is, anesthesiologists learn to trust it. I rested my gaze on the empty suction canister where blood would go if lost and felt something that lacked definition but I knew to be oppressive.

The patient's blood pressure dropped into the mid-70s systolic.

"How did you check her central line pressure?" I asked Nurse A.

Behaving as if insulted by my question, Nurse A shook his head while turning the stopcock that shifted the central line from intravenous access mode to pressure monitoring mode. The waveform signature of the patient's heart showed up on the screen along with the number 10 at the side. "See, I told you," he said.

I inspected the waveform and saw the problem. A central line waveform has several components, each component reflecting the action of the heart during a single heartbeat. True, the number at the side read 10, which is slightly above normal, but that number was the average of a very low number, reflecting the true filling pressure of the patient's heart, and a very high number, reflecting an artifact caused by the patient's incompetent tricuspid valve. Nurse A had failed to inspect the waveform closely or, more likely, didn't know the waveform's different components. He had simply taken the average number as gospel.

"She's bleeding. Her real central pressure is 1," I insisted.

"We didn't lose that much blood," the surgeon muttered to himself. But the warning whisper of sober reason had begun to counsel him. We all stared at the patient's abdominal wall. It had grown tighter during our short debate. The patient was bleeding internally.

Everyone sprang into action. The surgeon sliced through his suture line and inserted his sucker. Blood poured into the canister, sending great foaming breakers against its plastic walls. An ominous alarm on the blood pressure monitor rang. The patient's pressure had dropped to 60/35.

I injected a cardiac stimulant into the patient's central line. Her pressure rose to 85/50. But this slight movement upward was like an engine that had slowly risen up a long and steep ascent and was standing at the top, waiting for some master force to propel it forward and downward with irresistible force. Blood kept streaming out of the wound. The blood pressure monitor sent its alarming cries throughout the room. 81/49. 72/38. 61/21. We were going to crash.

During a crisis, everyone in an operating room begins to view life from a singular angle. The minds of all are suddenly concentrated and their bodies efficiently perform their assigned tasks. The surgeon worked furiously, sucking, cauterizing, and stitching. The operating room nurse called the blood bank and demanded that blood be made available for immediate pickup. The orderly raced over to get it. In three minutes, he dashed back into the operating room, panting heavily, as though fleeing an enemy, carrying a large white box with a red cross emblazoned on each side. Nurse A and I worked to place a second intravenous line in preparation for the massive blood transfusion.

Once the initial pool of lost blood was evacuated from the abdominal cavity, blood oozed more slowly from the patient's bowel. But somehow, somewhere, it found vent; it spirited up in a thick dark stream, submerging the intestines again. Looking for holes under such conditions is like trying to spot coins under murky water. Had the torn vessels been arteries, the job would have been easier, as arterial blood spurts and pulses with great force, leaving an obvious trail back to any vessel opening. But the operation had rent mostly veins, and each time the surgeon scooped out a handful of blood to look for vessel tears, another handful welled up out of nowhere and flooded the field. The surgeon could not find all the holes.

The patient's pulse was now barely palpable. Her white face was suffused with a blue tinge, her eyes rested wearily in their sockets, the lines underneath them darkened funereally. The process of disintegration had begun; the whole framework of the patient's existence had suddenly, in the twinkling of an eye, become a faded, shadowy thing.

Nurse A and I transfused the first round of blood products. I noticed the surgeon breathing heavily like a wounded animal, his body heat wafting upward toward the low ceiling. The patient's bleeding remained uncontrolled. I shot a glance at the monitors. No blood pressure was measurable. I expected the laws of nature to assert themselves any second, and for the patient's heart to give out too. Yet the EKG showed the patient's heart was still beating. The pacemaker had kicked in. Her heart was no different from a busted watch that keeps ticking by virtue of its battery. I injected epinephrine into the patient's intravenous to constrict her blood vessels and give her some semblance of a blood pressure. Thirty seconds later, 35/15 flashed on the screen.

The surgeon furiously sutured and cauterized. Nurse A and I squeezed four more rounds of blood products into the patient's bloodstream.

Her blood pressure rose steadily: 50/27. 68/44. 81/51. The surgeon grew less frantic. We were on an upward path. Thirty minutes later the patient was stable.

Such a right-about-face of destiny is common in anesthesiology. The patient's course moves swiftly toward disaster; then suddenly things are well again, a mischance prevented, a horrible outcome forestalled. Life, which suddenly seemed on the verge of being lost forever, belongs to the patient once more. But what brain damage the patient had suffered during the period of absent blood pressure we did not know. The surgeon resutured the abdominal wall. We hoisted the patient's bony body onto the stretcher and moved her to the intensive care unit.

I removed the breathing tube a day later. The patient suffered some weakness on her left side. She strengthened over the next week. After a month, she regained all of her function.

Who was responsible for this near catastrophe? The surgeon? After all, the surgeon had caused the bleeding. Yet if the patient's tissues were inherently friable and prone to oozing, no one could blame the surgeon for the blood loss that inevitably followed. Me? True, if I had done the case on my own, I might have noticed the drop in central venous pressure earlier. But a doctor today inevitably works with subordinates, and those subordinates must be free to make decisions. Indeed, subordinates rebel if not allowed such freedom. A doctor with experience knows that it is both impossible and counterproductive to micromanage the activities of every subordinate. A supervising doctor shapes the general direction of the case or points out certain general trends. The traffic officer regulates the flow of traffic; he or she does not assign a particular course to each car.

Nurse A? Closer. If Nurse A had alerted me to the drop in blood pressure before things had gotten out of hand, the catastrophe might have been averted. But that simply begs the question of why he had not. For that we must blame the medical profession.

Nurse A had internalized professional medicine's definition of the doctor as a master technician. Because Nurse A was technically accomplished, he grew cocky. Having mastered what he believed to be a doctor's core duties, it was only natural that he would imagine his capacity for doctoring to extend into other areas—such as managing the patient's sagging blood pressure on his own rather than alerting his attending. How doctors define themselves had initiated a cascade of events that almost led to a catastrophe.

It also explains why my first nurse anesthetist was so ill natured and intractable. She resented the salary differential between her and me—and naturally so, for if the medical profession tells her that a good doctor is a good technician, and she is a good technician, then all that separates them is salary, which to her mind is arbitrary and unfair. BSN, MSN's behavior was rooted in similar thinking. She saw doctors as her masters, and she liked being paid by her masters, but she wondered why she ought not to become a master herself, especially since well-trained nurses can insert needles and prescribe pills as well as any doctor can. Hence, the idea of "team medicine."

I encountered a variation on this attitude a month before writing this chapter. I was traveling on the highway. A car had crashed ahead of me. A paramedic truck was parked beside it. I stopped, got out of my car, leaned over the crash victim, told the paramedics I was a doctor, and offered to help. Rather than welcome my assistance, the two paramedics at the victim's side ignored it. One paramedic, with a scowl, asked me what kind of doctor I was. I told him I was an anesthesiologist. As the patient's face dripped blood, the paramedic shrugged and said, "I've probably seen a lot more trauma cases than you." His purpose at that moment was not to help the crash victim, but to make the point that here, in the field, he was more of a doctor than I was.

Nurses may protest. They will say I have generalized from a few bad apples to condemn all nurses. That is not my purpose. Moreover, any such generalization would be grossly inaccurate. Like most doctors, most nurses are hardworking professionals with a sense of balance about what they do and do not know. They take good care of their patients. They are knowledgeable and bring a wealth of experience to patient care. It is no surprise that the safest format for practicing anesthesia remains an anesthesiologist and nurse anesthetist working together, thereby doubling the trained set of eyes and ears around a patient. Doctors and nurses were practicing team medicine long before "team medicine" became a political cause, a catch phrase, and a movement. Few nurses are like BSN, MSN or Nurse A.

But neither are there many catastrophes. I would be remiss if I didn't place the correct interpretation on those few catastrophes that I have experienced in my career to benefit the reader from the lessons and, for that matter, the warnings they contain. We all know the ideal of the doctor and the nurse. But in this world of dreams, are we justified in ignoring the few nightmares?

5

WHEN PATIENTS BECOME CONSUMERS

A week later, while still new at the hospital, I was assigned to another D and C. My patient was nervous, and when she fretted that her surgery was scheduled for a full hour, I tried to reassure her. "Don't worry. It's more like ten minutes," I said.

Several days later, a senior doctor approached me with a grin on his face. "Did you tell that patient her surgery was only ten minutes?" he asked.

"Yes," I replied.

The doctor laughed. "Young man, never tell patients it's ten minutes, even if it is. When they get the surgeon's bill, they'll feel swindled. 'All that money for just ten lousy minutes!' they'll say. Always tell them at least thirty."

"Welcome to private practice," I joked sheepishly.

"Don't worry, you'll learn, but the surgeon is mad because his patient thinks she's been cheated," he replied.

Most doctors learn at some point that satisfying patients involves more than just curing them of disease. Patients always feel a little vulnerable in a doctor's presence. Nakedness threatens their self-respect; a physician's superior knowledge threatens their self-confidence; patients who would not ordinarily admit their weaknesses suddenly find themselves forced to discuss their most intimate problems, embarrassing them. Then there's the doctor's bill. On top of that, patients worry about being hurt with scalpels and needles. And, of course, there is the fear of dying. A curiosity in medicine is that upon disease—a very natural phenomenon—the most exquisitely complex emotional states are erected. For this reason doctors learn to treat patients somewhat gingerly and to accept their unreasoning sides. Nothing is stupider than the doctor who, from scientific or doctrinaire heights, is contemptuous of a patient's funny feelings and ideas.

Nevertheless, the doctor-patient relationship is an inherently unequal one, and the unreasonable patient who tries to make it equal—for example, by telling a doctor how to practice medicine—risks complications, even catastrophes. One might compare the impulses of a patient's mind to the movements of the ocean. One patient complains about his bill; a second patient complains that his doctor gave him bad directions; a third patient complains that her doctor didn't return her phone call. The wise doctor never becomes exasperated by such events. Like the mariner in a storm, he or she slackens sail, waits, and hopes; eventually, the storm passes and the voyage continues. But a patient who demands to be on equal footing with his or her doctor creates the conditions of a permanent storm, making travel dangerous.

I encountered this problem during my second month in practice when caring for a doctor's wife scheduled for a vaginal hysterectomy. I anticipated trouble upon greeting the woman in the pre-op area. I spied her coiffed hair and exact lipstick. Her wrists and fingers were adorned with gold. Her whole presentation seemed astonishingly expensive and well ordered, and out of place for a surgical theater. In those days being a doctor's wife meant something, and this woman wanted everyone to know she was no ordinary patient.

I told her it would be best if she wiped off her lipstick. She refused.

"All right, can you remove the nail polish from just one finger?" I asked.

"Why are you insisting on this?" she asked with inexplicable pride. "Are you always so rude to your patients? Or maybe you just don't like the color."

I knew what was going on. The source of her stubbornness was not in me but within herself. The woman felt vulnerable, and understandably so. She needed surgery on a bodily area that, to her mind, defined womanhood; she was scared and embarrassed; even her flirtatiousness sprung from fear. If a doctor analyzes looks, words, and gestures, and is open to hidden meanings, he or she can usually explain the rough treatment he or she is getting from a patient.

But this woman was interfering with my ability to take care of her. I told her I had to be able to inspect her skin color while she was under anesthesia, to check for anemia or hypoxia. She continued to resist, although in a sweeter tone. "Please, doctor, I'm just used to looking my best," she pleaded. Her emotion was a complex one, made up of pride, a claim to delicacy, an appeal to my willingness as a man to sacrifice my desires for a woman, and a need to establish self-assurance by winning a difficult victory. In any other patient I would have insisted on the fingernail polish (and the lipstick) coming off, but since she was a doctor's wife and a special case, I relented.

The nurses also relented by letting her keep her jewelry on. Indeed, the whole operating team was on edge because of her VIP status. They scurried around to create an exceptional surgical experience for her, an experience that fit her so well that it seemed as though the best doctors in the city had consulted among themselves how to proceed in the best possible fashion. When the woman arrived in the operating room one nurse fussed about her, putting a pillow under her head as she lay down. Another nurse stood at her side and held her hand. Lying on the table, her gown unwrinkled, her bracelets and rings shining exquisitely under the light, her body unruffled and still, the woman looked as if she had been chiseled into marble, the work of a brilliant sculptor—the perfect beginning to a perfect operation. And yet one of the nurses forgot to give her an antibiotic.

I gave the woman some narcotic and Versed. Rather than fall silent, she grew talkative. She confessed to having crush on the surgeon. The surgeon's eyes smiled at me; then he nodded his head—my cue to put the patient to sleep quickly before she said anything more embarrassing.

I would be remiss in writing a book about anesthesiology, even a serious book about anesthesiology and medical safety, without answering the question I am asked most often about the field: Do people talk under anesthesia, and, if so, do they ever talk about sex? Now would be a good a time to answer this question. Yes, people under anesthesia do talk about sex. In my experience, and in the experience of other anesthesiologists I've talked to, women talk more than men. I once had a patient blurt out under sedation the name of the man she was having an affair with. A second patient blurted out the name of the man her best friend was having an affair with. A third patient imagined aloud during a vaginal prep that she was having intercourse. A fourth patient mumbled during jaw surgery, "How long until I can have sex?" Her question confused the operating room staff, as her surgery wasn't gynecological, until she complained that her husband demanded oral sex, which she hated performing. She asked if she could have her jaw wired shut for a year to absolve her of the duty. I have many such stories.

Back to my narrative. I intubated the patient, turned on the anesthetic gas, and let the surgeon work. Now would have been the right time to wipe off the lipstick. Foolishly, I did not. On the contrary, I had been so careful not to smear it during the intubation that I was almost proud of myself. A few minutes later, the pulse oximeter (a probe placed on the finger to measure oxygen levels) malfunctioned—not surprisingly, since in those days pulse oximeters had difficulty seeing through nail polish. I fiddled with the device, trying it on different fingers, when I suddenly noticed that the pressure needed to push air into the patient's lungs was higher than expected. With the pulse oximeter malfunctioning and the woman's fingernails covered in polish, I instinctively glanced at her lips to inspect their color. They were bright red—from lipstick. I quickly wiped off the lipstick to reveal their true color, which was dusky because of a drop in oxygen levels.

I figured the breathing tube must have drifted too far into to the patient's right lung, causing the left lung to go without oxygen. I listened to the patient's chest with my stethoscope, confirmed the diagnosis, and pulled the tube back. With both lungs now oxygenating, the patient's lips pinked up immediately. The rest of the case went uneventfully, although when wheeling the patient back to the recovery room, I noticed a red furrow on her wrist where her bracelet sat, caused by pressure from the armboard against the metal. I kicked myself for not having insisted that she remove her jewelry.

This was not a catastrophe, but it might have been. It taught me something about doctors and patients.

Patients often do themselves a disservice, and even increase their risk of catastrophe, when they try to stand out. Doctors and nurses generally work best when allowed to follow their routines, and patients who emphasize their VIP status just throw everyone off kilter. Exceptions are made. Deviations from protocol are permitted. Duties are overlooked because everyone is anxious. Such patients often get worse care, not better.

From an anesthesiologist's perspective, it is often safest for the patient to have no identity at all. This goes against the grain of contemporary medical training, which tries to humanize doctors and strengthen their emotional connection with patients. Some doctors today even pride themselves on making friends with their patients.[1] A few doctors call such behavior unprofessional. But more important, it's dangerous. The more emotionally involved anesthesiologists are with their patients, the less they are able to think and reason during a crisis. The notion that someone dear to them, or to others, might die at their hands unsettles them. When disaster looms, they anticipate the tears on the faces of grieving family members, and fear spreads unreasoningly throughout the different compartments of their mind, clogging their reason. It is why an anesthesiologist is never supposed to put a family member to sleep.

Some of the finest anesthesiologists see patients as nothing more than bodies to be anesthetized. When waking up a patient from surgery, they scan the anesthesia record to relearn the patient's name before calling it out, and then just as quickly forget it. Nameless patients stop being VIPs or even individuals. Even a patient asleep on the operating table remains an individual if he or she has a name; the anesthesiologist imagines asking the unconscious patient a question and thinks to himself, *I know what he would say; if only he were awake, he would answer!* Patients with names stand out. VIPs stand out even more. Nameless patients do not. A nameless patient is just *human*, just a concept. The anesthesiologist experiences less fear when taking care of such a patient.

Callous, yes, but it lets the anesthesiologist's mind work methodically and correctly during a crisis. Good medicine is a fine balance between worrying about a patient and not caring at all.

The following week, I took care of a sixty-five-year-old man, Mr. D, scheduled for a trans-urethral prostatectomy (TURP). When he asked me about the anesthetic, I suggested spinal anesthesia. I told him there was no significant difference in mortality rates between general and spinal anesthesia, except when doing a TURP. It was the one operation where spinal anesthesia was recommended, as the anesthesiologist can more easily detect the unique complications of a TURP in an awake patient under spinal anesthesia. Mr. D didn't care. He demanded general anesthesia because he had heard that spinal anesthesia left people paralyzed. I told him how rare that was. Mr. D didn't care. I told him how a cluster of bad outcomes had occurred during the 1960s, in the United Kingdom, when glass spinal anesthetic ampules had been stored in formaldehyde to keep them sterile. Formaldehyde had entered through cracks in the ampules, paralyzing patients when the mix was injected into their spines. The tragedy hit the newspapers, I explained, causing spinal anesthesia to be unfairly maligned. Mr. D didn't care. He demanded general anesthesia and said it was his *right* as a patient to choose.

I understood his fears. He feared being paralyzed. He also feared surgery on his penis. Most men do. The very idea sickens them. Nevertheless, Mr. D's challenge signified a greater trespass on my authority as a physician and a greater risk of catastrophe than had my patient the week before. The doctor's wife had demanded an exception that interfered with my ability to monitor her under anesthesia. Mr. D wanted to decide the entire anesthetic.

Mr. D's demand didn't come out of the blue, especially his use of the word "right." Cultural change lay behind it. The patients' rights movement grew out of a larger bioethics movement that started in in the late 1960s, bringing the discourse of moral philosophy into the world of professional medicine. Words such as "rights" and "autonomy" spread from the university to the patient's bedside. The bioethics movement, in turn, arose from other rights-based movements, each with its own medical connection. The civil rights movement invoked the infamous Tuskegee experiment, where black men with syphilis were purposely denied treatment for decades. The women's rights movement rebelled against restrictions on abortion. The gay rights movement condemned psychiatry for calling homosexuality abnormal. Each of these movements had their counterparts in Europe, and each, in turn, drew from an even larger set of ideas, including the belief that medicine had become an oppressive arm of the modern industrial state.

But the pedigree of Mr. D's demand also included something uniquely American, as the patients' rights movement in the United States was also part of a larger consumer choice movement. By the 1970s, Americans no longer wanted to choose from among four kinds of breakfast cereal; they wanted to choose from among fifty. It was the same with cars, television shows, and every other kind of consumer product. Americans wanted the right to customize their consumer experience. This demand penetrated medicine in subtle ways. For example, drug companies, which had confined their advertisements to medical journals for much of the twentieth century, began marketing their products directly to patients—now viewed as consumers—starting in the early 1990s. This was unique to the United States, as drug companies are still banned from advertising directly to the public in Europe. This shouldn't surprise, as state-dominated health care—indeed, state-dominated anything—is often antithetical to consumer choice.

I hesitated to pick a fight with Mr. D. After all, some patients do have TURPs under general anesthesia without problems. Just because an anesthetic is suboptimal doesn't mean it's illegal. I also took the words "rights" and "autonomy" very seriously. I believed in the ideology. The problem was that Mr. D's urologist was mediocre. His urologist cut into prostates in ways that opened up channels for the glycine-filled solution used during the procedure to flood into the bloodstream. In addition, the surgeon was technically slow, made worse by his tendency to talk sports and politics. He would operate for thirty seconds, then raise his head to argue something about Democrats or Republicans, during which time more fluid would pass into the patient's system. That is why I wanted to use spinal anesthesia. Unlike a general anesthetic, which can theoretically last for days, a spinal anesthetic lasts only a couple of hours, which forces a urologist to quit cutting at a certain point, regardless of whether he or she wants to. In addition, I could detect fluid overload in Mr. D more quickly if he were awake.

But I couldn't tell Mr. D that his surgeon was lousy. Physicians have a code. When a layperson asks a physician to recommend a good doctor, the physician won't recommend someone terrible. But if a layperson is already under that terrible doctor's care, physicians usually avoid badmouthing that doctor to his or her patient, unless the patient is a friend or family member, in which case they tell the patient immediately. Mr. D was a stranger. I couldn't tell him that I needed to do a spinal because his urologist was slow, sloppy, and a chatterbox. So I let it go.

We brought Mr. D into the operating room. I induced general anesthesia and the urologist started working. Sure enough, every few minutes he launched into a tirade about Congress and, later, the National Football League. To prod him to return to work, I told him he had to finish quickly to lessen the time for fluid to enter Mr. D's bloodstream. "Oh, yeah. Sure," the urologist replied in agreement, but then a short time later he moved his head away from the cystoscope and started talking again. He was in the mood to talk.

I should have been more adamant in telling him to shut up and work, but politics intervened. In those days, surgeons often behaved like kings, expecting not only to be obeyed but also to be entertained. Some of them saw the anesthesiologist as a kind of court jester, to speak to them when they desired conversation, to shut up when they didn't, and to grovel before them when they wanted to feel important. Anesthesiologists were once happy to perform in this role, since surgeons brought the patients, and without patients there would be no work. "Yes, it's embarrassing what we're doing, trying to humor the surgeons," anesthesiologists would admit to themselves. "So long as we remain fully conscious, it's for the good of the practice, it's okay. Just don't make a circus of the job." Rather than protest when the urologist talked, I was soon giving my own opinions on the national debt and the likely winner of the next Super Bowl.

About ninety minutes into the procedure Mr. D's blood pressure climbed higher. No change in anesthetic state or surgical stimulus explained the increase. I assumed it was from too much fluid entering the patient's bloodstream through the open prostate, so I told the urologist to move things along. He refocused, only to lose his way again.

"Who do you think will win the next election?" he asked.

The patient's blood pressure rose higher. Had Mr. D been awake, I might have been able to glean important data from his complaints. Shortness of breath would have suggested fluid overload. Restlessness, confusion, and nausea would have suggested water intoxication. Gradually, the inflation pressure needed to push air into Mr. D's lungs increased, most likely from fluid overload. The urologist had to stop.

"That's enough. You're done," I said sternly.

"Just a little more. Really. Maybe another twenty minutes," pleaded the urologist.

"You said that twenty minutes ago. No, you're done. If you have more prostate tissue to shave off, you can bring him back another day. He's showing signs of fluid overload," I insisted.

The urologist glared at me but quickly wrapped things up. I turned off the anesthetic gas. Twenty minutes later Mr. D was still unconscious. We brought him to the recovery room. I ordered a blood test for a sodium level, which came back 119 (the normal is 140). It explained Mr. D's sleepiness. Too much sodium-poor fluid had entered his bloodstream through the open prostate sinuses. Indeed, the sodium level was so low as to risk seizures. Yet I couldn't treat Mr. D aggressively with sodium because that would have expanded his blood volume when he was already fluid overloaded and risk pushing him into heart failure.

After five hours, the sodium returned to acceptable levels. Mr. D woke up—blind. It was a known, albeit rare, complication of TURPs. Glycine in the cystoscopy solution had entered the patient's bloodstream in large amounts, interrupting neural transmission in his retinas.

"I can't see!" screamed Mr. D.

I tried to evaluate Mr. D's vision, but he kept shaking his head in panic. "I can't see!" he screamed.

His eye exam was consistent with glycine toxicity. I stared at his sightless head, feeling helpless. I tried to explain to him that his blindness was likely temporary, but my words of reassurance were drowned out by other sounds in the recovery room, all bombarding his consciousness.

I sedated him with Versed, hoping his vision would return by the time the drug wore off. He woke up an hour later. His face was as blank and lifeless as the faces of the blind. Then he cried. I gave him another dose of Versed. When he woke up an hour later, he saw light but no forms. I tried again to reassure him, but other sounds from the recovery room kept coming, flying, falling over one another. A clamorous darkness. They tortured him. He started to cry again. I gave him more Versed.

Two hours later, he woke up and said he could see vague forms. He was calmer now, in part from the Versed but also because he sensed things were improving. He still had that far-out gaze. Over the next hour, more images filtered their way to the dark recesses of his brain. He looked around to test his vision, reaching out to the recovery room's brightly lit parts. Increasingly, he enjoyed the conviction that he had seen. Two hours later, he did see.

I swore I would never let myself get into such difficulty again. In the future, if a patient refused my advice, I would refuse to do the case. Simple as that. After all, some doctors don't even give their patients a choice. "You're going to get a spinal. No discussion," is how one senior doctor said he would have approached Mr. D. I wasn't ready to go that far, but I was ready to shut things down if a patient demanded an unsafe anesthetic. Brave I would be to shut things down, I thought.

Then again, how brave would I be to shut things down simply because I feared telling my patient that his or her surgeon was mediocre? Not very brave. Something was missing from the oath I had sworn.

The courage to say "no" is a part of being a doctor. But it is only a part. A doctor also has to be flexible. He has to know what is possible. The sense of what is possible includes the ability to recognize that certain things are impossible—in other words, unsafe—but also to know that things that appear to be very difficult are in fact possible. A stubborn patient can sometimes be charmed, coaxed, nudged, or inspired to follow the wiser path. A good doctor does more than just draw red lines and say, "No." He or she also persuades.

It is the difference between commanding and governing. To command is to lead a group of people under discipline toward a clear goal. A general commands a group of soldiers. A dictator commands a whole society. Both expect to be obeyed. To govern, however, is to lead people toward unclear and shifting objectives, with nothing really compelling people to obey.

A doctor governs rather than commands a patient. A patient is not compelled to obey a doctor. When a patient is healthy, he or she is even less likely to obey. A doctor also has other constituents, including a patient's family, nurses, and other doctors, all equally free. A patient's family is not compelled to obey a doctor. Officially, nurses are compelled to obey, but, unofficially, they will push back if doctors use the wrong tone with them. Other doctors are no more compelled to obey a doctor than a patient is. The impulses of these free people—patients, patient families, nurses, and other doctors—are at all times a parallelogram of forces. They are hard to synchronize. A doctor must know what these forces are. Sometimes he must say to himself, "I can go just so far and no farther"; he must say "no" and refuse to do something he thinks is unsafe. But he must also have a sense of what is possible; he must calculate how much he can move one party without offending the others; he must foresee the inevitable reactions of the other parties when one party is appeased; he must always be taking the temperature of the various parties to see if one party's willingness to compromise has bled into anger, hurt feelings, and obstructionism.

Just as a governor is careful not to appease one class at the risk of angering another, a good doctor should not shield another doctor at the expense of his patient. Yet this must be done tactfully, with finesse—to keep the parallelogram of forces from working at cross-purposes. If I could do it over again, I would tell Mr. D in the pre-op area, "Your urologist is a very thorough surgeon and takes longer than average to perform a TURP. So it would be safer for you to have a spinal." It might have done the trick. Mr. D might have been nudged onto the safer path, while his urologist would have been spared direct criticism.

All this may seem trivial, silly, and even slippery. But in doctoring, as in politics, it is useless to formulate grand theories of human relationships if, due to the parties concerned, they are irrelevant. Doctors know how to make polite bows to theories of human behavior to appease those who guard temple gates. But doctors actually occupy themselves with taking care of people's real needs. If they find obstacles, they make detours; if they encounter resistance, they cajole, sweet talk, finesse, and even play games. The true doctor says, "Let the principles go and save the patient."

A year ago (and twenty-five years after taking care of Mr. D), I attended a conference on a new concept in medicine called "patient-centered care." Its purpose is to give patients and their families more say in their medical decisions. Although I went to the conference to investigate, I met an anesthesiologist from out of state who had been compelled to attend. She told me her story.

She had come in on her day off to take care of a morbidly obese twenty-five-year-old woman needing gall bladder surgery. The patient had requested her. She met the patient and the patient's father in the holding area. The father insisted that he be allowed to accompany his daughter into the operating room to hold her hand while she went to sleep. He also insisted that she be given gaseous anesthesia before receiving an intravenous, as his daughter was afraid of needles. In regard to the first request, the anesthesiologist told him that bad things can happen during an anesthetic induction, and that a parent's presence can interfere with a quick response.[2] Exceptions are made in cases involving children, the anesthesiologist said, but not in adult cases. In regard to the second request, she told the father that a gas induction in an adult increased the risk of serious complications, including loss of the airway and death—especially in morbidly obese adults. It's much safer to use a conventional intravenous induction, she said. Despite her reasoned arguments, the father refused to back down. They argued back and forth. Finally, the father gave way, but later he complained to the hospital administration about his "mistreatment." He was especially angry that the anesthesiologist had called his daughter "morbidly obese," although this was the official diagnosis according to medical terminology. (Morbidly obese is defined as twice one's ideal body weight.) Instead of supporting the anesthesiologist in her decision, the hospital, which employed her, reprimanded her and gave her a Wikipedia article on patient-centered care. They said the patient and her father were "customers," and that her job as an employee was to satisfy them. They ordered her to attend a conference on the subject, issuing vague threats about what might happen if she didn't.

We entered the conference room together. Doctors from all over the region were there. Four panelists sat on the podium: a Stage IV breast cancer patient, a hospital administrator, a doctor, and a nurse practitioner (with the ominous appellation "BSN, MSN" after her name).

The breast cancer patient spoke first. She talked about how, when diagnosed with metastatic cancer, a surgeon had given her only one option, a mastectomy, not to cure her but to give her a little more time to live. An equally narrow-minded oncologist had recommended only chemotherapy. "This is what I give to all my patients," the oncologist reportedly said. When asked if there were other options, the oncologist said, "Nope, that's it."

At this point, something between a hiss of detestation and a murmur of horror ran through the audience. The woman then talked about how she explored other options on her own. She finally decided on palliative care so that the time she had left wouldn't be filled with the painful side effects of chemotherapy. "It's important that *consumers* be given all their options," she concluded. "They are when buying cars, so why not in health care?"

The woman was sweet and sincere. And dying. The audience reacted sympathetically. I was surprised that such arrogant, close-minded physicians still practiced. Why not give a breast cancer patient all her options? Even as a medical student in the 1980s, I was taught to do so. In that respect, patient-centered care seemed like another variation on the old patient autonomy movement that began in the late 1960s. Still, I was surprised to hear patients called "consumers."

The hospital administrator followed. He spoke more as if reading out an indictment. Doctors were charged, collectively and individually, with gross insensitivity to patients and their families, refusing to accommodate patient wishes and needs, refusing to give weight to patient opinions, and covering the traces of their crimes with appeals to science, claiming that science guided their behavior when, in fact, it was arrogance, dictatorial tendencies, and a lack of empathy. He cited Dr. Donald Berwick, former head of the Centers for Medicaid and Medicare Services, who had spoken recently at his daughter's medical school graduation about a woman who had been denied access to her husband's deathbed because of physician policy.[3] It had been "cruel," said the hospital administrator, which was the same word used to describe the incident in Dr. Berwick's speech. The administrator added more incriminating stories—for example, a doctor's refusal to pray with a nervous patient before surgery. Finally, having piled up all the evidence he required, the administrator smiled triumphantly and pronounced a new age of patient-centered care, an age of "transparency," "dialogue," and "inclusion," in which patients would no longer be "marginalized."

The audience remained silent. No one thought of presenting the other side. No one was even sure if there was another side. Personally, I didn't disagree with the administrator, although his language disturbed me. I smelled ideology. "Marginalization," "inclusion," a more "just culture"—these were all catchwords of the political left. And why the revolutionary fervor? The patient autonomy movement had already been around for forty years.

Next, the doctor on the panel spoke. He described a YouTube video that had gone viral and showed doctors and nurses dancing in the operating room as the patient entered. Apparently the patient was nervous and to ease her fears had requested not only that music be played but also that the staff dance to it. The audience chuckled. This seemed a bit over the top. We assumed the speaker was reassuring us with an example of the new policy's outer limits: true, in the future, doctors would have to be more flexible in the face of patient demands, but they wouldn't actually have to go to such ridiculous extremes. Instead, the doctor on the panel praised the video as an example of good patient-centered care.

I think the audience and the speakers at the podium understood each other at this point. A fundamental shift in the power relations between doctors and patients was under way. Patients were consumers now, and the doctor's job was to give them what they wanted no matter how ridiculous their request seemed. It only remained to present the new concept in PowerPoint form, to dress it up in its proper ideological clothes, and to link the talks of the four speakers into a more or less coherent whole.

The doctor went on to confess how he had ignored patient desires in the past. During this part of his speech he seemed to shrivel and contract. His shoulders were hunched, his head bowed. If the panel had wanted to convey what they believed to be the grotesque past of doctor-patient relations, they could have chosen no better means than this penitent fig ure. After confessing his crimes, the doctor talked about the future. Doctors, nurses, and patients would all be on the same "team," he proclaimed. Doctors would embrace "patient preferences and values" rather than ignore them. Doctors would be "advocates" for their patients. His words reeled off like a well-learned lesson. Indeed, they almost seemed to be delivered as if he were under the influence of some drug or hypnotic spell. His statements didn't really add anything new to what the others had said; in fact, they were altogether superfluous. Nevertheless, he was a doctor who had given a confession, and one sensed a ripple of satisfaction passing through the other panel members. Having played his part, he sat down and fell silent.

Finally the nurse rose to speak. After declaring her deep passion for patient-centered care, she admitted that doctors must follow the standard of care when practicing medicine. "That's paramount," she said with confidence. But doctors also had to integrate a patient's values into their decision making, she declared. "Standard of care and patient needs are never mutually exclusive," she insisted.

I looked over at the anesthesiologist whom I had walked in with, hoping she might tell the room about her case. I raised an eyebrow when she looked back at me, as a cue for her to speak up. Instead, she privately waved me off. I was not surprised. She had come to the meeting to learn correct thought and to clear herself of the slightest suspicion in the eyes of her employer. The last thing she wanted was for her hospital to hear that she had been difficult.

So I spoke. While leaving her name out, I described her case, focusing on the dangers of breathing down a morbidly obese adult with anesthetic gas before placing an intravenous.

"In this case the standard of care and what the patient's father wanted *were* mutually exclusive," I concluded. "The standard of care should have trumped patient desires in this case, correct?"

There was a stir of interest in the audience.

The nurse stared at me and declared, "No, they are never mutually exclusive. In the case you describe I'm sure a compromise was possible."

"But it wasn't," I replied.

"It always is," the nurse shot back.

"But in this case there wasn't. The father refused to budge," I said.

"I can't imagine that. I can't even consider that," insisted the nurse.

The entire panel looked annoyed. They were not used to someone in the audience declaring opposition to the new program. They also knew I was saying things that, for some physicians, might not be without their attractions.

Another anesthesiologist in the audience spoke up. "Breathing an adult down with anesthetic gas is not actually a breach of the standard of care," he said.

The panel members seemed to relax for a moment. I caught the nurse's eye and found her regarding me with a significant smile, as though to say, "You slipped up."

"But it is a breach of the standard of care in obese patients," I countered. "Such patients have a much greater risk of aspiration,"

The other anesthesiologist said nothing in response. Yet no one else in the room backed me up. Even the anesthesiologist whose case I cited remained silent. I felt alone, like the last survivor of a vanished race—doctors who value safe practice above any other consideration.

Another doctor tried to effect a compromise: "Can we at least say that patients with special wants and needs should contact their surgeons or anesthesiologists in advance, so there will be time to accommodate them?"

"That's a good idea," replied the nurse, hoping this would end the exchange.

But I refused to remain quiet. "In the case I mentioned, the father's desire expressed in advance wouldn't have changed anything. Breathing down his obese daughter with gas would still have been dangerous," I said.

"There was a way. There was a way," replied the nurse, angrily. "The doctor involved in your case could have done something. He probably just refused." Deliberate sabotage on the part of a doctor was somehow a much more satisfactory explanation to her mind than a doctor's desire to follow practice guidelines.

I disagreed. This time the nurse sought refuge in generalities. "Listen, medicine used to be a one-way street, with doctors telling patients what to do. Now, it's going to be a two-way street," she said, with a note of scorn in her voice.

The hospital administrator piled on. "That's right. It used to be that the doctor was in the front seat, driving the car, while the patient was in the back seat. Now, the patient is going to be in the front seat, too. Not necessarily in the driver's seat, but definitely in the front seat," he said.

These were nice metaphors, but they bore no relation to the reality of the case we were discussing. I said so, and then harped again on the rules governing anesthesia safe practice.

The nurse grew angrier. The hospital administrator adopted a more self-satisfied expression. He was the kind of businessman who is obstinately sure of himself and thinks only he sees the big picture. He laughed sarcastically as I spoke. "Some rules are important. But other rules are silly. Everyone knows that. Sometimes you have to break a silly rule. You can let the hospital know if there's a silly rule. We'll make a note of it," he replied.

"But what if a doctor thinks a rule isn't silly? And what if the doctor breaks that rule, gets a bad outcome, and gets sued? What's the doctor supposed to do then?" I replied.

The physician on the panel shifted uneasily in his chair. From some last remnant of professional pride, or from some strange feeling of honesty surviving all other emotions, he quietly said, "That's a good point."

The nurse glared at him. He fell silent, back to whatever limbo he had come from.

Instead of answering my question directly, the nurse sidestepped it. "If you and a patient have issues, just call for a mediator on staff," she said.

"Is the mediator a doctor?" asked a physician in the audience.

"Sometimes the mediator is a nurse," replied the nurse, defensively.

"So we're supposed to let a nurse decide what is best, and the doctor is supposed to accept the nurse's ruling as final? That doesn't make any sense," said the physician.

Other doctors spoke up. They finally had a glimpse of the meshes in which they might be entangled themselves one day. One physician took an altogether separate line, aiming it directly at the hospital administrator.

"How can you tell us to spend more time with patients to learn their needs while also telling us to keep our office visits under ten minutes? How can you tell anesthesiologists to take time to meet patient needs while also telling them to start their cases on time or be penalized?" she asked.

A few in the audience murmured in approval. More debate was imminent. But for the nurse and the hospital administrator things had already gone too far. The nurse was wedded to her idea of patient-centered care, and she seemed worried that more debate would threaten her chance to transform that idea into reality. The hospital administrator, however, was more interested in practical considerations. Hospital surveys had shown that patients wanted patient-centered care. Several hospitals had already toyed with the idea of setting up patient-centered floors, where inpatients and doctors share completely in decision making. Patient-centered care was going to happen whether the doctors wanted it or not.

The hospital administrator implied that all dialogue was now at an end. "Listen, I know people fear change. That's natural. But what you fear now you will get used to eventually. I remember when doctors once feared the concept of informed consent. They thought it was crazy. Of course, it wasn't. And doctors got used to it," he said with feigned lightheartedness. "Just as you will get used to patient-centered care," he added in a more threatening tone.

Bit by bit, the fantastic structure took shape in my mind. I began to see how patient-centered care differed from the old patient autonomy movement that had tripped me up twenty-five years before when caring for Mr. D.

Mr. D had demanded certain rights as a patient. In the years to follow, patients became even more demanding, especially when they gained access to medical information through the Internet. The patient autonomy movement in the United States was always especially strong.[4] Many doctors grew to resent their patients second-guessing them. Yet, as a whole, the movement proved to be a good thing, protecting patients and giving them a needed say in their care. Moreover, a stable equilibrium grew up between doctors and patients over time. Patients learned more about their treatment options and had more say in their care; when patients pushed too hard, a doctor could always say, "I can go just so far and no farther."

But a consumer rights component always lurked within the patient autonomy movement. It is not just as *patients* that people today want control over their care but also as *consumers*. This is the energy source behind patient-centered care. In fact, Dr. Donald Berwick, a leader in the

patient-centered care movement, writes in his manifesto that patients today are "consumers" who should have "choice in all matters, without
exception."[5]

Not surprisingly, the patient-centered care movement is stronger in the
United States than in any other country America respects and values
customer service; it is an integral part of the national character. American
politicians and clergymen play upon the feeling of respect for service as
much as businesspeople do. Politicians call themselves "public servants,"
while the church performance itself is called a "service." The compelling
spell of patient-centered care is hard for any American to resist—even
doctors.

The patient-centered care movement does have the potential to
achieve its own stable equilibrium, just as the patient autonomy movement did. Yet an unrelated trend in American medicine makes this hard to
achieve, raising the risk of catastrophe: doctors in the United States have
increasingly become dependent employees.

Most doctors once worked either as self-employed professionals or in
small professional partnerships. In the last fifteen years, more doctors
have become employees of large institutions, such as hospitals or corpo-
rations. With dependent employment come bosses and the fear of being
fired, especially for not giving customers what they want.

Doctors today feel pressure from both above and below. If doctors
make their patients happy, they can keep their jobs; if not, they risk losing
them. Doctors feel enough fear that some of them will adopt a risky
course to please their customers. In one example I am familiar with, a
doctor at a hospital in the southeastern United States acceded to a patient's demand that she be allowed to hold and nuzzle her baby immediately after delivery during a cesarian section and while still on the operating table. The anesthesiologist thought it unwise, as the patient was at
high risk for postpartum hemorrhage, but she felt pressured by the hospital to give the mother what she wanted. She allowed the mother to hold
her baby after delivery. When the mother suffered a serious hemorrhage,
the baby's presence prevented the anesthesiologist from easily accessing
the mother's intravenous. The nurse wrested the baby from underneath
the mother's gown, but this took time, during which the mother lost
consciousness and possibly aspirated, as her oxygen levels remained low
in the post-op area. Fortunately, she made a full recovery.

A situation analogous to what has happened in medicine has happened in academia. Students today see themselves as consumers, especially given the high price they pay for college. Sometimes they demand that professors tailor their lectures to please them, even if that means learning less. Yet professors only found themselves at risk of losing their jobs when college administrators, who technically employ them, agreed that students were customers, since they were paying the bills, and therefore should be given what they wanted. It was only when professors realized they had bosses, and could be fired for failing to satisfy their customers, that they felt pressured into giving in to students.

In academia, the stakes are a student's education. In medicine, the stakes are a patient's life. Sandwiched between employers above and customers below, doctors are fast losing the ability to say, "I can go just so far and no farther."

6

A TALE OF TWO OFFICES

A man today goes into a hospital and feels himself lost in some great city. No one takes any notice of him. If he asks for directions, busy staff bristle with irritation or ignore him altogether. He wanders along a corridor, telling himself, "When this corridor comes to an end there will be something pretty or heartwarming, or at least different, or maybe just space for my eye to roam," but no—there is nothing but another corridor like the one he has left, and whether he looks to the right or to the left, he sees corridors and rooms, all alike, over and over again, closing in on him like an army of robots. No interesting sight for his eye to rest on, no stained glass windows, no crown moldings, no fireplaces. Nothing to inspire him. No real space or even a sense of imagined space. The man feels hemmed in on all sides—and his thoughts and feelings are hemmed in too.

The mid-twentieth-century Catholic hospital where my father worked as a doctor had a different air. It functioned as a hospital but looked like a church. Cherubs, angels, and garlands were carved into the white stone edifice. Wide steps at the main entrance led to a heavy wooden door with black iron hinges, with the door itself contained inside a Gothic arch. The peaked roof over the entrance supported a large white cross. Inside the building, the halls were dark and foreboding. Here and there, slanting beams of sunlight passed through small windows and picked out from among the shadows the faded pictures of Christ that hung upon the walls. In this dim world, Catholic sisters in white habits glided about solemnly from sickroom to sickroom, in a somber yearning for divine intervention that scratched at their belief in an omnipotent God, while visitors sensed that irrational forces were at play, and that mankind was not totally in control. A hush fell about little children as they walked around, many of whom steered close to their parents out of fear. Even drug reps entering the building on business felt tempted to bow their heads.

As a child, I often went on rounds with my father. Whenever I entered the hospital, leaving the hot California sun behind me, a black cloud would suddenly weigh heavily on my brain. There was the smell of damp air. The hall was inexplicably cold and dark. And quiet. A profound respectful silence reigned, except for the chapel music that quailed with a painful sigh, and that made me feel melancholy. My father would take me onto the wards to greet his patients. The rooms were full of terrifying diseases, or so I thought. A creaking noise from a door would send shivers down my spine, as though a monster inside had moved. On the walls hung pictures of terrible heavenly wrath: a writhing Jesus, a fiery ball over Sodom, locusts causing famine, and the deeply furrowed face of God.

In this world of permanent twilight I saw through my child's eyes what I believed to be fantastic creatures.

I saw a doctor wearing a clean, long white cape (what I later learned was an operating room cover gown). I imagined that cape flowing backward as the doctor flew through the sky. The doctor flew over peaks and precipices, flinging thunderbolts at disease; were it not for his brave schemes and brilliant exploits, a terrifying death, a death that frightens the imagination, would descend upon all. Dare one doubt a doctor's powers? Why, when he approached certain doors they magically opened because he commanded them to. Sometimes they only opened halfway and stopped, as if to taunt him, and then the doctor would stare back angrily, and they would open up completely, unable to withstand his power. (I later learned these were electric operating room doors.)

I also saw a beautiful creature clothed in a white dress and white cap. Tender, sweet, and kind, she was the nurse. I compared her soft hands with the doctor's cold, sharp instruments. I worshipped her graceful pride and light step, and the delicacy with which she mopped a patient's brow with cool compresses. She would lean over and pat the patient's pillow, and the patient would shake with pleasure, his sensitive nose smelling the clean scent around her neck, the fragrance of lemons, of fresh air, of the country. Then she would clean the patient, comb his hair, take his temperature, and ask him how he slept and whether anything troubled him. Sometimes her medicine hurt, and yet even if she inflicted pain by giving the patient a shot, it was a kind and helpful pain! The pain was over quickly, and then the nurse would stroke the patient's head and cry with him (if he were a child), and even if the patient threw a tantrum, she would go on being nice to him.

I saw a doctor's wife in the distance. So regal! The queen of the realm. And yet so busy. Family happiness and the care of the hospital were her sole business in life. At the hospital, she would volunteer and spread good cheer. She worked in the gift shop. She baked pies for the nurses. I often picked through the cart of magazines and knick-knacks that she pushed around the wards. Yet the doctor's wife was more than just a street peddler. She kept a wary eye on all that went on in the hospital and her husband's office. When a patient complained about the cafeteria food, she saw that it was fixed. When the hospital needed a new machine, she put on a pretty dress (not without pride) and charmed her friends into giving money. On the hospital board she was always consulted. Her home life was just as much a continuous dashing and scurrying around. She never complained because her husband came home late at night, or because a sick patient ruined the family vacation. She cooked supper while the children played around their father, climbed on his knees, and put their arms around his neck. After dinner she made sure the children did their homework so that one day the white coat would pass from father to child, just as it had passed from grandfather to father. Later, while her husband snored away upstairs, she would pore over office receipts, clicking the keys on the adding machine, and not until she finished would she go upstairs and fall soundly asleep.

I glimpsed another woman behind a counter. With her white headdress, her diminutive size, her large twinkling eyes, and her white, almost translucent skin, she looked like a mythical fairy creature peeping out trustingly from behind a giant oak. I wondered if she was winged, like an angel. No, she was a Catholic sister. Her whiteness and purity reminded me of the nurse; yet she was not motherly so much as transcendent. Shining brightly, she would come over to me, take me by the hand, and say her holy words—a prayer so beautiful that I thought it should be accompanied by a lute. A smile of happiness would spread across my face, and I would think, *The doctor will fix me, the nurse will love me, and the sister will bless me.* As in fairy tales, I imagined her keeping evil spirits imprisoned in enchanted dungeons, her words depriving them of any ability to harm me. When she finished her prayer she would stuff me full of candies that were hidden inside in her habit. Then she would withdraw gradually, as though reluctantly, like the sun drifting down toward the horizon, only to return and bring her warmth another day.

Beloved hospital of old! Your memory, a remnant of a dream of the historic past. It rises amid the gray monotony of the present day—dim, misty, tinged with the sweetness that breathes from memories of the vanished past. Vanished—yes, but not without a trace! It still lives, this past, in wards where sick patients lie worrying and search in their imaginations for something to ease the fear of what encompasses them. It lives in legend. Low I bow and kiss your tender shadows, hospital of old. I kiss your mythical inhabitants, cavalcade of honor, your chapel's rapturous song of the nightingale.

My grandfather was born in a small farming village in Germany in 1893. His father was a cattle dealer. Beginning in 1912, he studied medicine in Munich for a year, then Freiburg for another two years, and then Frankfurt for two more years. Such hopping around was common among medical students in those days and reflected nothing more than a desire on my grandfather's part to see some nice towns. He served in World War I (on the German side) as an auxiliary field doctor before marrying my grandmother and settling down in Frankfurt to work as an internist.

Times were hard. Germany almost starved during the first few years after the war. My grandparents lived on horseflesh. The prescription pad saved them, as milk was available by prescription only, so my grandfather could get some. With extremist politics adding another layer of uncertainty, my grandparents emigrated to Washington, D.C., in 1923. Once there, my grandfather set up a practice on Columbia Road, within walking distance of Garfield Memorial Hospital.[1]

Life became easier. Nevertheless, my grandfather's medical practice failed to take off. Anti-Semitism wasn't the problem. On the contrary, Garfield Hospital had a long history of welcoming Jewish physicians. The first contributions to build the hospital actually came from two small Jewish congregations, the news of President Garfield's assassination having reached them on the Hebrew Sabbath. Nor was the problem a lack of friends. My grandparents had busy social lives. Still, none of their friends ever became patients.

At first my grandparents took the problem in stride. On rare days when my grandfather actually brought home money, my grandmother would tease, "You've got the *gewinnthosen* on" (in translation, "winning pants" or "money pants"). My grandfather would happily use the downtime in his office to read German literature and philosophy, sitting cross-legged in a cloud of cigar smoke, his favorite pastime. Fortunately, my grandfather's brother, a Washington department store owner, died in 1935 and left him some money. But this only slowed the drift toward disaster.

My grandfather's problem was that he couldn't adapt to the new American conception of the doctor that had taken hold a decade before.

In the first half of the nineteenth century, the United States faced an emerging physician surplus, as almost anyone could call himself or herself a doctor. By the second half of the nineteenth century, American doctors were required to have actual training, but a glut of medical school graduates left the United States with twice as many doctors per capita as in England and four times as many as in France or Germany. At root, it was a physician identity problem, with four competing schools of thought over what a doctor should be. One school, exemplified by Dr. James Jackson, cofounder of the Massachusetts General Hospital, said the doctor was a gentleman. Another school, personified by Dr. Jacob Bigelow, said the doctor was a technician. A third school, associated with education reformer Abraham Flexner and the new Johns Hopkins University Medical School, said the doctor was a scientist. A fourth school, personified by Rev. Henry Spalding of Chicago's Loyola University, said the doctor was a benefactor. Each cluster of schools churned out graduates, flooding the country with doctors and adding to the confusion. In 1910, the Flexner Report on Medical Education ended the debate by giving rise to a new vision of what a doctor should be. This new vision was a compromise of the four schools. Henceforth, an American doctor was part gentleman, part scientist, part technician, and part benefactor.[2]

My grandfather failed in each category. As a scientist, he had fairly decent medical training in Germany—in fact, one of his professors was Röntgen, the discoverer of X-rays—but he didn't *look* like a scientist. Most American doctors had switched over to wearing white lab coats by 1915, to advertise their connection with science. My grandfather, however, continued to wear a dark suit, as doctors had in the nineteenth century.

The suit made him look like a clergyman or, worse, a mortician. Prospective patients didn't like it.

My grandfather's office compromised his credentials as a technician. Most American doctors' offices were well-planned complexes by the 1930s. They included a reception room, a private office and consulting room, a dressing room, a business office, a room for physical therapy treatments, and an examination room. The examination room, in turn, usually had an examining table, a stool, a floor lamp, an instrument cabinet, a scale, a sink, and a waste receptacle.[3] My grandfather's office was just one room. Instead of an examination table, it had a low-lying twin bed. There was no stool. To perform a pelvic exam he would ingloriously bend down on his knees and then struggle to raise himself up afterward. A weak overhead light substituted for a floor lamp. The instrument cabinet was poorly stocked and in disarray. The only sink was in the bathroom. None of this suggested technical competence.

The wooden desk and chair standing in the office corner gave prospective patients another reason for pause, as did the wooden floor. The American public had learned the basic principles of antisepsis by this period. Prospective patients expected medical office furniture and appliances to be made of metal, often with white enamel coating, to allow for easy cleaning. They expected floors to be linoleum for the same purpose. The wood in my grandfather's office was hard to clean and often stained. Worse, wood was a living thing, like the germs themselves.

My grandfather was an intellectual and not a gentleman—failure again. He was astute, but his astuteness often degenerated into profundity. He liked to talk to patients about German philosophy even when they didn't want to listen. He also loved mechanical order and would exhibit an almost mystic fidelity to a plan, making him rigid and inflexible. He was the stuff out of which idealists are made, but also autocrats. Prospective patients thought him "too German" or simply weird.

True, my grandfather was a benefactor. He often took care of patients for free or overlooked their unpaid bills. It is one reason why the family finances were in such a precarious state. But my grandfather misunderstood that to be a doctor-benefactor in the Land of the Dollar, he was supposed to be a businessman without appearing to be a businessman. The American doctor's job was to feign a lack of interest in money while making money all the same.

My grandmother was poorly equipped to help him. Because the AMA had erected a ban on physicians advertising, in accordance with the ideal of the gentleman-doctor, doctors had to be less direct in how they drummed up business. Many physicians relied on their wives to gain them patient referrals. At Garfield Hospital, auxiliary organizations were staffed with doctors' wives who worked to improve the hospital (their husbands' place of business, after all) but also to connect with other wives to influence their husbands' referral patterns. My grandmother had no such social acumen. She had been educated to be the wife of a *German* doctor, not an American doctor. She knew how to dance, play the piano, and cook. She could rush to answer the phone and, with dignity, say, "Let me see if 'the Doctor' can speak with you," or "No, 'the Doctor' cannot speak with you." She could tell the neighborhood children to keep quiet, declaring, "There's a doctor upstairs who needs his rest." But that was all. Her psychology was even less suited to business. She lived on her nerves; she was quick in emotion and sentiment, a prey alike to hopes and suspicions; she was excitable, but without an excitable person's saving store of common sense.

By the late 1930s, my grandparents were close to losing their house. One day, my mother, then a young girl, went with her father to help him clean up his office. He sat in his wooden chair and cried.

"I'm sorry. I guess I haven't been a very good doctor," he said.

"Oh, Daddy, it's okay," my mother replied, trying to reassure him. Old urine bottles sat on the cupboard behind her.

"I'm sorry. I'm sorry," my grandfather said repeatedly, his eyes moist.

Fortunately, things ended well. A friend who understood my grandfather's personality found him a salaried position as a physician at the Old Soldiers' Home in Washington, D.C.[4] By the standards of the day, my grandfather was a failure as a doctor. The AMA saw "salaries" as an acceptable method of payment for common laborers or civil servants but not for gentleman-benefactors. Nor did my grandfather have an office in his new position. But he did have access to examining rooms with proper examining tables and linoleum floors. He could take care of patients without having to hustle for a living. He could be himself and talk German philosophy to old American soldiers, who were now his captives. He was even given a white lab coat to wear, in homage to science. To friends and family he became a doctor in full.

Twenty years later, my mother was vacationing at a Catskills resort. It was the last day of the season. Lying on her lounge chair at the end of the afternoon, she watched an ugly woman make one last trip around the pool to catch a man's attention before heading into the locker room. It was the woman's last chance, her last plea for companionship, my mother thought. But none of the men looked at her. On the trip's final leg my mother observed the woman's crestfallen face and the silver strands in her hair. My mother decided that she herself had better get married quick. A month later, while working as a lab technician, she met my father. They married the following year, on April Fools' Day. But the joke was on them.

Hitler once said that the war in the west, between the Germans and the British, was a war of conquest, while the war in the east, between the Germans and the Russians, was a war of annihilation. And so it was with my mother, the German Jew, and my father, the Russian Jew: their marital fights were not mere spats, or even shouting matches, but wars of annihilation. Each tried to destroy the other. Being a busy doctor, my father had no need of excuses to keep away from home, thereby postponing the decisive moment, but both knew that one day the moment would come, that they would have to divorce, although each was equally hesitant to make the break, for their own reasons, even if each knew the break must come.

One evening in the early 1970s, my father arrived home just as my sister, her boyfriend, and my sister's school friend were teasing me in the living room. I was thirteen. My sister was fifteen. Her boyfriend was often at the house, usually bringing his big dog with him and tying the creature up to a sprinkler pipe outside. My father hated both the boyfriend and the dog. As for my sister's school friend, southern California's culture of sex and drugs had aroused an unhealthy curiosity in the girl when she was twelve; by the time she was fifteen she had the air of a dissolute, much too experienced woman. All of us grew up uncontrolled.

"Come here and kiss my cheek," my sister ordered me. When I complied, she squealed, "Ugh! So wet! No girl's ever going to want to kiss you." Then her friend led me over to a mirror and maliciously said, "Kiss the mirror until you get it right. There should be no wetness on the glass."

For five minutes I dutifully did as I was told, until my father came over and asked me what I was doing. I naively replied, "They said I don't know how to kiss, and that if I don't practice, the girls won't like me."

"Do you want the girls to like you?" my father asked me.

"Well, I don't know," I replied, uncertain and confused.

My father rolled his eyes. With a cynical, world-weary tone of voice, he said, "Well, when you do, just wag a dollar bill in front of them."

My mother overheard the comment and grew angry. When my father sat down to dinner—alone, as the rest of us had already eaten—she reached into the oven for two lukewarm burnt lamb chops that had been cooked that afternoon. She put them on a plate, along with a scoop each of soggy mashed potatoes and canned peas, and thrust the food in front of him as if he were a dog.

"Here you are—choke yourself!" she said to my father. She went back to clean the counter with an expression of disgust.

"I work all day and this is all I get?" my father shouted.

"Maybe if you made more money, you could wag a dollar bill in front of me. You might get a better dinner," she hissed.

"I make enough money. A lot more than your father did. He was a—"

"You shut up about my father!" my mother interrupted.

"You shut up! If you threw some parties and got me more patients, I'd make more money. Why can't you be like the other doctors' wives?" His face grew as red as beetroot. "You lie around all goddamn day like a martyr, telling me how tired you are from playing tennis!"

"You're the one who told me to take up tennis!" my mother protested.

"So you could meet people and throw parties!" my father shouted back. Then he proudly declared, "I'm doing well enough. When my new office opens I'll be doing even better."

"I'm sick of hearing about your damn office!" my mother shouted.

"Well, I'm sick of you!" my father yelled back.

"Fine, go ahead and build your glorious office," my mother said sarcastically. She paused before delivering her knockout blow. "A real big deal, you think you are. A Jew with plans, a Jew with ideas, a Jew who thinks he's going places. Ha!" she sneered in a mocking tone, looking at my father through the derisive slits of her eyes.

A spasm of rage clutched at my father's throat. He threw the dinner plate on the floor and stood up, while my mother's face grew increasingly purple and distorted. Suddenly the live-in Mexican maid walked into the room. Her presence worked like a cadmium rod in a nuclear reactor and brought the two people back from the brink of explosion. My sister, her friend, and her boyfriend dashed into my sister's bedroom and slammed the door behind them. I remained behind and turned on the television.

A pleasant warm breeze streamed westward from the desert, reinvigorating the well-trodden grass around our driveway. In the air hovered the never ceasing buzz of bees and the metallic ringing of sprinklers. The smell of honeysuckle mixed with the acrid scent of seawater. Quartz crystals embedded in our house's facade glittered in the sun.

Inside, while waiting for the party guests to arrive, my father went over the plans for his new office. He had already purchased space in the professional building. The complex was to have four examining rooms, an X-ray suite, a laboratory, a lavishly decorated waiting room, a business office, a wood-paneled private office with an ocean view, a consulting room, a library, three bathrooms, and a kitchenette. The furniture was to be all Duncan Phyfe.

The new office was my father's dream. It went hand in hand with his dream of being a doctor. Like my grandfather, my father loved being a doctor. But unlike my grandfather, my father's sense of identity as a doctor was perfectly in sync with the American ideal. As a nod to science, my father always wore a white lab coat in his office. Indeed, he owned six white lab coats. As a nod to technology, my father always kept his stethoscope in his coat pocket, and always so that it was visible, even on days when he knew he wouldn't need the instrument, because he believed it was part of the doctor's uniform. Also, my father had specialized and become a hematologist. In his role as benefactor, my father gave free care to the poor and never advertised (even after physician advertising became legal in 1975), but, unlike my grandfather, he hustled, building himself a nice independent practice. In his role as gentleman, my father talked with patients without lecturing them (as my grandfather had). He was also discreet with patients, sometimes even a little mysterious and impassive, radiating a polished aloofness that he had purposely acquired over the years to keep patients at a distance, and that patients seemed to appreciate, as it made him seem like a doctor and not just any person off the street.

Small things, but to my father they summed you up as a doctor.

The décor of his new office was impregnated with all these themes. The office was to have a library of medical journals, complete with back issues, to remind patients that there, in science, lay the springs from whence medicine drew its strength. The examining rooms were to have the latest equipment, each machine so beautiful that nothing else was needed in terms of decoration. Indeed, the chastity of the technical style worked on the principle that the essence of the thing not be spoiled with anything extraneous; the machines were the objects for which patients came, so it made sense that only they be there. The waiting room, by contrast, was faux European gentleman, evoking a blend of old manor house covered with ivy, transoceanic steamer, and Versailles, and purposely conveying to patients a sense of solidity and gravitas. When talking with patients in the similarly furnished consulting room, my father would be as a landed proprietor, walking over his estates and talking with his tenants, learning the real state of feelings and needs.

What the office was *not* was a tribute to money. Some business offices are explicit tributes to money, more specifically to the cleverness, boldness, and ruthlessness that created the fortunes that made the offices possible. Such offices awe people while also reminding them of the elemental unfairness in life. My father's office strove for the opposite feeling, to carry people on wings into a world where money is secondary and to lure them away from capitalist thoughts with allusions to distant times and places where thoughtful benefactors once existed.

My mother was conflicted about the new office. On the one hand, she took her identity as a doctor's wife as seriously as my father took his identity as a doctor. She volunteered regularly at the hospital. She felt like an important personage when patients muttered under their breaths as she passed by, "You see that lady? She's a doctor's wife." Sometimes she would go to the hospital early, leaving me to get to school on my own. (As a nine-year-old, before I could tell time, the end of a particular television show was my cue to depart when my mother was absent.) My mother also appreciated a nice office. But the memory of her father's office sometimes pulled her in the opposite direction. She admired her father, and if a shabby office was good enough for him, it was good enough for anyone, she thought. Still, she did admire success.

She also feared that my father wouldn't get enough patients to fill all those new examining rooms, and that his investment would go south. She knew my father. She knew he was weird. His jokes were often corny or silly. He once showed me a slide presentation that he was preparing for the local medical society. Inserted between two slides of medical data was a slide of a naked young woman lying on the beach. "Now how did that get in there?" Dad laughed with mock surprise. When I asked him why he had put that slide in, he quipped, "Wakes up the audience." Nor was my father a back-slapper. He liked classical music more than sports. The other doctors blackballed him from their local fraternity. To make matters worse (and unbeknownst to herself), my mother was also weird. She had a wicked sense of humor that scared the other doctors' wives, putting a limit on how much she could coax them to get their husbands to refer cases to my father. None of this prevented my father from building a medical practice and making a good living. But filling four examining rooms with patients, all day, every day, was a stretch given both my parents' personalities.

The guests started coming up the walkway, all doctors and their wives. I was inside the house, lying belly down on the orange-red shag carpet, vigilantly watching television. I heard a dog bark, then the front door swing open, followed by a loud "Hello!" but my eyes never left the screen. A minute later, I overheard one guest telling her husband, "That's the Dworkin boy."

"Hello, Ron, how are you?" she asked me.

"Okay," I replied, without turning my head.

"Where's your mother?"

"Outside."

The woman tried to engage me in conversation. "Your mother told me that you're going to be a doctor, just like your father. Is that true?"

"Yes," I replied reflexively, my eyes still glued to the screen.

"Are you going to be an internist like your father?"

"Yes," I replied, without moving my head.

From the other side of the room, I heard the screen door slide on its rudder, followed by a torrent of words that made me shudder.

"Quit watching television and go swim with your sister!" my mother shrilled with her special mixture of affection and anger, although I also detected a sliver of anxiety in her tone. I picked myself up off the carpet and slinked toward the backyard, incapable of offering her any opposition.

I jumped into the pool. My sister and her boyfriend were kissing each other in the deep end. More guests arrived. Every few minutes I would reach for the tray of potato chips and onion dip, tasting the tang of onion, salt, and chlorine on my fingers as I listened to the conversation around me.

"You have to raise your rate every year, regardless of whether the insurance companies pay it," I overheard an older doctor telling a younger one.

"Why?" the younger doctor asked.

"That's how you keep up your financial profile," said the older doctor. "Even if just one insurance company pays your rate, you can tell the other insurance companies, 'See, this is what I'm getting. If you don't pay me my rate, then at least pay me close to it.' And raising your rate is good for all of us. It keeps the financial profile for the whole region high."

My mother, another doctor, and his wife were talking about my father's new office.

"I hear your husband is building a new office," the doctor asked my mother.

"Yes," my mother replied with a snide tone of voice. "That's all he ever talks about. As for me, I could care less." Instinct caused her to look over toward my father. With a nervous chuckle, she added, "Oops, I think he overheard me. See? He's looking over here with his big bug eyes." She left to go talk to my father. I listened to more conversation.

"It's quite an office, I hear," said the wife.

"Is he breaking through a main wall?" the doctor asked with real interest.

"I think so," the wife replied.

"Well, then, it really is a big project. Where did he get the money?" the doctor wondered.

"I don't know. At any rate, someone doesn't spare expense," the wife said.

My father was angry because they had run out of ice. He yelled at my mother as she clawed for cubes in the most remote corners of the freezer. "Damn you!" he whispered to her, hanging over the top of the freezer door.

My father had no choice: he had to ask my sister's boyfriend to go to the store for more ice. "Sure," the boyfriend replied dumbly. "I'd do anything for you guys. I love your daughter." My father grimaced. The boyfriend hopped on his motorcycle and sped away. Ten minutes later, he revved up his bike's engine to announce his return, his dog barking and competing with the bike's stuttering, backfiring roar for my father's attention.

An hour later my father noticed the party was also short on dessert. Again, my father yelled at my mother, but this time he went to the store himself. When my father returned, the boyfriend's dog, which had been sunning itself on a patch of ground, leaped up and fastened its teeth on my father's pant leg. My father howled and thrust the dog off with his free hand. Endeavoring to keep to his feet, he dragged himself toward the front door. He stumbled into the house and poured out a torrent of angry words at my mother.

Later that evening, after the guests had left, my father yelled at my mother about my sister's boyfriend, the dog, and the botched party. The screaming was horrible. "Close the window, or the neighbors will hear," my mother said. My father purposely opened the window even more and shouted into the world, "I don't give a goddamn if the neighbors hear!" My mother returned fire. Finally, my father declared, "That's it! I'm leaving!" Driven at full speed toward an act predetermined in the depths of his consciousness, and for over a decade desired in his heart of hearts, he raced into the bedroom and emptied his drawers in three armfuls, placing everything onto the bed. Then he opened his side of the closet and snatched a large suitcase he had been storing for just this moment. He threw his clothes and shoes into the suitcase, closed it, and grabbed four suits on their hangers.

"Where are you going?" my mother asked.

"To find happiness," my father answered.

From behind, my mother shouted caustically, "Find happiness? Good luck! It's the same everywhere, stupid!"

My father stormed out of the house. From the open doorway, my mother shouted, "Why are you leaving? Just because your daughter has a damned boyfriend?"

Leaning out his car door window, the gray Buick Riviera gliding slowly in reverse down the driveway, my father declared, "I'm leaving because killing would be too good for you!"

Life changed little for my mother. A week after my father left, she played tennis with another doctor's wife while I sat nearby on a bench. The two women rallied for thirty minutes, then played a set. My mother was the better player and should have won, but she lost on purpose (she later told me) to butter up her opponent. Afterward the two women and I sat down to lunch.

"Everything okay?" my mother's opponent asked her. "Seemed like you were struggling out there."

"It's a difficult time," my mother replied, sounding melancholy. Then she explained how my father had left the house.

"No! Really?" the tennis partner asked.

"Yes, it's true," my mother uttered despondently.

"That rat!" the tennis partner declared.

"My life is lousy right now," my mother declared in a high nasal wail. "It's unfair, isn't it? My children are fatherless, I'm left all alone, but his life is untouched."

"We'll see about that!" the tennis partner shouted.

Within three months my father had lost 20 percent of his patient volume. Each of his referral sources gave him the same explanation: "It's not me. It's my wife. She's mad because you walked out. She won't let me send any patients your way—and she works in the office, so she'll know!" Even the Catholic sisters at my father's hospital, who often received phone calls from patients asking for the name of a good doctor, and who would suggest my father, stopped referring to him. "Awful, isn't it?" they reacted angrily. "Such a nice family, with three beautiful children, and he just ups and leaves."

A month later, my father could take no more and returned home. On his first evening back he crawled out of his car and walked toward the front door. The dog belonging to my sister's boyfriend was chained to a pipe nearby. The dog snarled at him, straining at the leash, eager to bite into his flesh. The animal turned back only when my father opened the front door. Upon entering the house my father heard my sister's bedroom door slam shut, then the pop of his own bedroom door being banged closed. He went into the kitchen and made dinner for himself. He ate the meal slowly, blinking moodily. I was engrossed in watching television ten feet away and never once bothered to say hello.

In southern California, a hamburger isn't just a *thing*. It's like a flag or the Bible. It has spiritual value. The smell itself forms an inescapable background to life in the region, quite unlike anything smelled elsewhere, a composite of various odors inextricably mingled with one another. There is the scent of burned fat and fresh buns. Add to this the aroma of warm asphalt and burned gasoline, and the odor of pool chlorine and ocean water, which somehow cling to the hamburgers as they're served. Given the high density of hamburger shops in southern California, the pleasing, pungent flavor pervades the entire region.

About a year after my father returned home he took some of the Catholic sisters and me out for hamburgers. He would often take the sisters places—for example, to concerts or to the opera—in part to stay on their good side and to keep the referrals coming, but also because he truly liked them and thought it a nice gesture.

I got to know several of the sisters over the years. One tiny sister in charge of the chapel would waft from room to room like a feather, her little nose scrunched up in a big smile. Her massive headpiece seemed unwieldy for her, as her whole upper body swayed in whatever direction the headpiece leaned, making her look more out of this world than most sisters. Another sister loved professional football, and she would pass me newspaper clippings of her favorite players. She admired a good tackle or a rush up the middle, but when she described them her words rang with a tender tinkle. A third sister grew up Baptist in the South, later converting to Catholicism. Her spectacles magnified her round, brown eyes, giving her an open and honest look, while the crucifix around her neck swayed in the air whenever she bent down to clasp my forearm with her soft hand. A fourth sister wore on her habit an image of a crown of thorns dripping red blood. She often took long walks around the hospital, which was in a bad neighborhood, and therefore dangerous, but the bloody crown was probably her best protection, as young hoodlums assumed she was the den mother of some violent gang, with the crown as its logo, a hint of the gruesome fate that awaited them if they dared to attack her.

My father both liked and needed the sisters, and he had good reason to keep them happy. The sisters, in turn, had good reason to keep the doctors happy, since the latter brought patients to the hospital, and they routinely fawned over them. A doctor would enter the hospital through a special entrance. There, every morning, he would be greeted with homemade rolls and donuts, fresh-squeezed orange juice, and butter rolled into little balls. A doctor could take as many buns as he wanted, then sit down on a plush sofa chair and with his free hand pick through the various news-papers and magazines lying on the coffee table, all neatly arranged by a sister before dawn. More food made by the sisters would follow him around the rest of the day—to the dictation room (the sisters' way of coaxing him to keep his charts up to date), to the conference room, and to the special room in the cafeteria reserved for physicians, which also served free homemade soup.

My father and I walked into the convent to pick up the sisters. For the first and only time, I saw its insides, including a small eating area. The cleanliness, the absence of clutter, and the small plates for small portions all spoke of the absence of men in the sisters' lives. The sisters moved around slowly in their habits. It was hard to imagine any of them having once run around in a child's body, young and well.

But some of the sisters did have mischievous spirits. On the way to the restaurant one sister wore a new soft headpiece, and she was glad about it, complaining that the hard one had kept her from driving all these years. It wasn't against the law, she said, but the Department of Motor Vehicles had told her it was dangerous. The hard headpiece had also kept her from eating a hamburger because the tight band under her jaw cramped her mouth, keeping it from opening wide enough to get the hamburger in. "I haven't had a hamburger since before I was a Catholic," she half-joked. She also said the hard headpiece left a permanent crease on her forehead.

We arrived at the restaurant and ordered. Everyone was so happy with expectation that it seemed almost sinful. I imagined the devil himself back in the kitchen, roasting the burgers on the grill. I imagined the grill with myself frying on it, blistering hot, flames all around, the oil scorch-ing my skin. A shiver went down my back.

I asked the sisters more questions. I asked them if they ever had birthday parties. They said the sisters held a party for another sister only on her namesake's feast day. Since a sister's old identity evaporated once she took her final vows, her actual birthday was ignored. I asked them if they ever went swimming. They said the company that made their habits also made special bathing suits for them. I told the sister with the soft headpiece that I liked it better than the hard one. The sister laughed, "I do too. Those hard ones make us look like creatures from outer space. They scare people. I try telling them not to worry, and that we sisters don't just grab anybody we bump into. There's got to be some sin involved. But that just makes them more afraid. You'd think I was going to shoot them with a ray gun."

The half-pound cheeseburgers arrived five minutes later, diapered in wax paper to dam up all the drippings. One of the sisters stared in astonishment. She could have never fit one into her mouth wearing the old stiff headpiece, she said. She crossed herself hastily so as to separate herself from animals who simply grub for their food in the wild. Another sister picked up her cheeseburger gingerly, as though it might explode.

In between bites I asked the sisters why some of them wore long habits and others wore shorter ones, above the ankles. The sisters grew silent. Something about my question seemed to bother them. One of them said it was just the fashion, and then she quickly changed the subject.

Years later, I discovered that the shortening of the habits, along with softening of the headpieces, the two weeks' vacation that some sisters wanted, and the right to live outside the convent and the right to serve a visitor a cup of coffee without getting permission from the Mother Superior, were all hotly contested issues among Catholic sisters during this period. Even Pope John Paul II had weighed in, attempting to reverse the trend toward disintegration in America's convent communities by reemphasizing the importance of wearing the habit, living in the convent, and practicing the vow of obedience. The sisters were living a centuries-old system of life, but for the first time they were doing so self-consciously; they were looking at their lives from the outside, scrutinizing them, judging them, thinking them hard and a bit unfair, and for this reason the whole system was rotting and waiting for the jolt that would bring it all crashing down.

Both the medical profession and the Dworkin family household faced analogous threats.

The following year, in mid-September, a hot, dry, boisterous Santa Ana wind blew down from the mountains. The thirsty earth steamed. My hometown was like a furnace, and one spark in the dry scrub would have set the whole city aflame. Dogs and cats moped across the bare and unhappy asphalt. A puddle of rust-colored water on the sidewalk seemed to them like an oasis. Outside the professional building that housed my father's new office, a flag flapped violently on its pole, sounding to passersby like a great chained bird beating its wings with all its strength, desperate to get away.

My father and I were on the sixth floor surveying an examination room in his new office. The machines were beautiful to look at. The EKG monitor, the diathermy machine, the blood pressure monitor, the scanner, the microscope, the incubator, and the X-ray machine—all were nickel-plated and streamlined; some sat on special polished platforms. The control panels had only a few buttons to press. Machines simply decorated, but on closer inspection therein lay their distinctiveness. Here were machines for the rest of your life, machines for the average man, machines for princes. *Never will these machines be out of fashion*, I thought. *Never will they grow old, just as diamonds and emeralds never grow old.*

My father walked over to his new waiting room and smiled proudly at the furnishings. A dignified lamp sat atop a cherry wood stand, the legs of which meandered gracefully toward a Persian carpet on the floor. Fine red leather sofas and chairs dotted the rugscape. Enormous ficus plants sat in white marble pots with gold handles. On the wallpaper hung several elegant paintings with ocean themes, along with a few cozy works painted by my sister when she was nine. My father saw real handiwork in his decorating; some doctors might even want to study with him, he said. He almost seemed to regret that his work, which really ought to be placed on public view somewhere, was instead going to be seen only by a small group of people with leukemia and cancer.

My father was smiling for another reason. Although his home life was as bad as ever, something had changed. He couldn't quite put his finger on it, but he had noticed that doctors' wives had less control in directing their husbands' referrals. Something about the new insurance system, something called "managed care," where bureaucrats now decided where patients went. Doctors' wives had lost power in other ways. He had heard about a recent hospital board meeting where a businessman had discussed ways to improve the hospital's finances. When a doctor's wife suggested improving the food in the cafeteria (which had always worked before), the businessman laughed with derision and dropped fancy abbreviations that no one had ever heard of, such as PPO, HMO, and ERISA. Then he mocked the poor woman, announcing to the room that the quality of the chicken in the cafeteria no longer drove health care.

In the past, for financial reasons, my father had been too afraid to leave my mother. But now, standing in his waiting room thinking about how much he loved medicine, but also how he had used medicine to divert his mind from his hatred of my mother, how he had thrown himself into the task of building a beautiful office, how he had moved the furniture about personally, and yet every evening, as soon as the bustle of the work day had subsided and the time came to go home, the mere thought that there, in the bedroom, like a vulture on a grave mound, sat my mother, frowning and terrible, causing him to feel weak in the pit of his stomach and all his energy to go out of his movements . . . yes, while thinking all this he was smiling. He knew he had the courage to leave.

My father and I returned home an hour later for another party. The doctors and their wives began to arrive. My sister was already treading water in the pool. The sun stared stubbornly in the sky.

I overheard snippets of conversation.

"Did you hear what happened to [some doctor's wife] last week?" the first woman asked a small crowd.

"No, what happened?"

"She was home alone when a burglar came through the side door. She fled upstairs to the bedroom and got out her husband's gun. The burglar followed her upstairs, and she shot him in the leg! Can you believe it? There was blood all over the marble floor, the police raced over . . ."

"What? They have marble on the second floor?" a second woman exclaimed.

The first woman telling the story looked stunned by the response, but others followed the second woman's lead.

"I'm surprised," a third woman said, turning up her nose. "I didn't think her husband was that successful."

"I'm sure a rich relative helped them," added one of the doctors.

"Helped them how? Paid for the marble floor?" interrupted the second woman.

"Most likely."

"I don't know," a fourth woman said. "They're adding on, I hear. I don't know if a relative would pay for an addition, too."

Life tensed thirty minutes later when a divorced woman walked through the door. She had been the wife of a very successful doctor, his practice a well-stocked hatchery from which to refer patients at will. My mother often imagined herself a queen, but this doctor's wife, she had once told me, was the "queen of the queens." That was all over now.

Although there was no longer any business reason to invite this woman, my mother had done so out of pity.

Some of the other guests were less welcoming. Before her marriage, the divorced woman had been a nurse. As a doctor's wife she had vaulted to greater status. After the divorce she had gone back to being a nurse—and in those days inviting a nurse to a doctors' party constituted a major social breach. Although doctors and unmarried nurses stood firmly with one another on the wards, their social lives never mingled, and neither the doctors nor their wives thought unmarried nurses were entitled to such equality. Indeed, at all the parties my parents threw or that my parents took me to, I never saw an unmarried nurse at any of them except this one time. A nurse had to be married to a doctor to attain the necessary social rank.

Many of the guests were rude to this woman. The doctors shunned her. Some of the wives feared her, for she reminded them of what might happen to them some day. They treated her the way pack animals abandon a wounded comrade in the forest. Other wives gloated, their body language saying, "Ah, girl, you failed in life." Already the party atmosphere was muted. In southern California, a Santa Ana wind drives people to water, but it also drives them apart; it makes life unmerciful, and people start to care only about themselves and how to get cooler. The presence of the divorced doctor's wife made the party atmosphere that much more sullen.

That night my parents had another fight. It was so loud that one of the teenagers next door yelled, "Shut up!" from over the fence dividing their house from ours. The party had been a failure, but I don't think either of my parents cared about that anymore. "I'm sick of these people!" I heard my mother shout. The next day my father moved out for good.

Finished, the comforting thought passed through my mind.

Two years later, my father's medical practice was in deep trouble. He didn't have enough patients to pay for his overhead. The office lease alone was killing him. The insurance industry's new dominance, in the form of managed care, was the problem. It affected not only how much doctors were paid but also whether they had any patients at all. And managed care had powerful allies, especially in government. Federal legislation had earmarked millions of dollars for the development of managed care. Later, in 1982, California state government would make enrollment in a managed care program mandatory for all Medicaid patients. Meanwhile, the federal government had removed all barriers from managed care's involvement in Medicare. The very mechanism that had allowed my father to leave my mother spelled doom for his career. He had gained his freedom, but at the price of a world.

Other doctors were in the same boat. And not just doctors were affected. The Catholic sisters also felt their power ebbing away. Once in charge of their hospital, they increasingly ceded control to professional businesspeople (often men). When Catholic sisters brought up their long-standing commitment to the community, businesspeople were usually milder in their criticism compared to their treatment of the doctors' wives. They said the sisters, at least, remained a "useful marketing tool" for the hospital. Yet the old business model—build a professional office building, entice doctors to come, pamper them, worship them, give them their own room in the cafeteria to dine in, and they'll bring the patients— was dead. It didn't matter if the sisters put a doctor's office in the middle of the chapel; patients weren't going there unless the insurance companies let them.

My father was despondent, but on this particular day his troubles struck him like a piano falling from an open window and crushing him to the ground. Once a year, his father (my grandfather) came out to California for a visit. The man had emigrated from Russia to Canada in 1912. To make a living he had owned a small candy shop. He had never finished high school, while his wife, already dead, had been illiterate. This man was incredibly proud of his son. During his visits to California, he would put on his best suit and go sit in the waiting room of my father's office, all day, and gaze at the beautiful furnishings, feeling himself to be somehow connected to them. Whenever patients came in and sat down, he would find a way to strike up a conversation with them and talk to them about their problems, and then tell them that his son was their doctor and would help them. There was something magnificent and touching in the pride of this old man, worn out by hard work and life in general, yet ready at any moment to tell someone that his offspring was more than just a speck of dust in the universe but, on the contrary, a son who had made good. My father knew how his father felt about him, and the actual truth of his situation tore at his heart.

That evening my father took me to a meeting of the local medical society. He was already in a bad mood. The topic of discussion was "managed care."

We got off the freeway and drove west along the street toward the hotel where the meeting was being held. Upon arriving, I noticed anxiety on the doctors' faces. Managed care threatened them all alike. In their daydreams some of them gave managed care a face, picturing it in their minds as a one-eyed giant marching across town, grabbing doctors, choking them, squeezing them to death with its cold, unfeeling fingers.

I heard snatches of conversation going on around me.

"Managed care is taking over everywhere," one doctor moaned.

"Where did you hear that?" another doctor asked through a mouthful of donut.

"I read it in a magazine," the first doctor replied. Then he added, "And they say nurses are going to be running everything. No more doctors."

"So what do we do?" asked the second doctor, still chewing.

"I don't know. But we have to fight."

The guest speaker was an insurance company executive trying to get the doctors on board with the new order. Tall and immaculately dressed in a gray suit, with fearless blue eyes, he looked like a colonel, and before uttering a word he posed in a picture-postcard attitude, his arms crossed, his face expressing great confidence, as if preparing to give orders with the expectation of being obeyed. His whole presentation was an indication of the insurance companies' might.

He outlined the present situation, touching briefly on rising medical costs, the inability of employers to pay their insurance premiums, and the problem of the uninsured. Playing to the crowd, he criticized and mocked the very idea of socialized medicine. Then he outlined what he called "the third way"—managed care—that would preempt government intervention, although it would alter how doctors organized their practices and got paid. This part of the speech was quite technical, filled with such terms as "preferred provider," "capitation," and "point of entry," and it confused the doctors, almost as if on purpose. Many of the doctors in the room grew suspicious. Although only a few of them could grasp the details of what the speaker was saying, they sensed the main thing, which was a threat to the old ways of doing things. Almost immediately there was a shout:

"Explain to us about 'capitation'!"

Hardly had the speaker finished his complicated explanation when another shout arose:

"We don't understand what you're talking about. We're not economists here. Use simpler words."

A howl of scorn arose from the assembly. The speaker's head turned this way and that, studying the doctors attentively and waiting until they were quiet. His first feeling of certainty that the doctors would welcome managed care to escape the threat of socialized medicine had passed, and, realizing the doctors' mood, he knew that a serious fight loomed.

A doctor in the audience attacked him in a personal way, telling him that he knew nothing about taking care of patients, that empty words were coming out of his mouth like soap bubbles, and that all he really cared about was making money. The insurance executive shot back vauntingly, and with a scornful look, that doctors wanted to make money, too. The doctors in the room fell silent; some of their faces clouded over. For the first time in their lives they had seen an insurance man who dared to insult a doctor in public. Used to deference from businesspeople, they stared back in astonishment.

The speaker left the podium. As he passed by, the doctors glared at him, while he, in turn, hid his disdain for them behind a smile. Afterward, the doctors herded together into clusters to share their contempt and apprehension with one another.

They could be broken down into three groups according to their shade of panic.

The first group consisted of foreign doctors who were born in authoritarian countries, had fled to America as adults, and were afraid of politics. Habitually passive in the face of conflict, their instinct was not to fight but to pray. Many of them wore gold chains around their necks, not to show off their wealth, but because in their home countries troublemakers were often jailed or shot; a person might have to flee at a minute's notice, and gold chains were a proven way of bribing a border guard. These men came to America to live in peaceful obscurity, to make as much money as possible, until the moment the authorities told them they couldn't make any more, at which point they would steal away with whatever loot they had and thank the authorities for sparing their lives. They were easy to spot in the large room, not because of their accents, but because they looked like mice, the way their eyes darted and glanced, and their whiskers twitched, suspiciously sniffing the air and looking around the room carefully, as if to check for the presence of a cat.

The second group consisted mostly of American-born doctors. Unlike the doctors in the first group, these doctors wanted to fight managed care. But how to fight? By what means? These doctors had long felt superior to businessmen, and yet now, when faced with a real threat from businessmen, they were flummoxed. Although each of them had more than a decade of advanced education and considered themselves privileged members of the American elite, they were incapable of intrigue, having never learned it, and even if they had learned it, they would have been averse to using it, having long had a feeling of fastidiousness about conflicts over money and power. These doctors were educated, successful, and polished; yet in some ways they had never really progressed beyond childhood—they spoke fighting words, but they were incapable of clenching their fingers into a fist and striking.

The third group included both American-born and foreign-born doctors. Shrewd men, they felt all the pulses of life and understood politics. They knew how to fight and how to hit hard, but they also knew when to fight, especially those doctors from authoritarian countries who had learned by experience. Had they been faced with such a crisis back home, they would have carefully maneuvered themselves into positions of power over the doctors in the first and second groups, not through bluster, but rather through strategy and cunning. Like the other doctors in the room, they hated managed care, having grown rich on traditional fee-for-service medicine. But they did not have the same self-satisfied arrogance about being doctors as doctors in the second group. On the contrary, rather than feel contemptuous toward businessmen, they saw themselves as businessmen; whether to fight managed care was purely a financial calculation on their part, and not a question of defending the medical profession's so-called honor. Since managed care appeared inevitable, some of these doctors were actually thinking of giving into it, joining it—now, before it was too late—with the goal of running the whole thing in five years.

A doctor from the second group went up to the podium to speak. He was tall, white, and elegantly dressed, in his late sixties, wearing a navy blue suit, a white cotton shirt, and an Ivy League tie. With his chest held high, he declared:

"We don't want managed care. It only brings shoddy medicine. And we won't allow a bunch of businesspeople to take care of our patients, to make a mockery of the Hippocratic Oath, and to desecrate the sanctity of the doctor-patient relationship."

The hall broke into thunderclaps. Handsome despite his years, with his hair a distinguished gray, his posture erect, and his face expressing determination and pride, the speaker looked like a leader. He went on:

"We have to stand together and fight, not negotiate. I'll never sign a managed care contract." The audience clapped again. It did their hearts good to look at him. He was an icon, not a doctor. Several shouts were heard:

"To hell with managed care!"

"Keep things the way they are!"

The speaker continued, many in the audience staring at him in admiration, even envy. He was elected to chair the committee responsible for fighting managed care. Around eight o' clock, the meeting broke up and all the doctors left the room, many of them confident that their fate had passed into good hands, that this distinguished, elegantly dressed man with the erect posture would destroy managed care and they could go back to business as usual.

My father also seemed reassured, as he always had had a feeling of fluttering respect for WASP physicians. But for some reason, while driving home, his confidence left him and he began to panic.

"My God," he moaned, "how everything changes. I finally have my office, and now this trouble comes along." Then he yelled at me, "What's the name of that fancy college you want to go to?"

"Swarthmore," I replied.

"Well, it's too expensive. Who do you think you are? The Prince of Wales?" he snapped. Then he returned to his own problems, and sighed, "What's the point of it all? Maybe nothing matters . . ."

He dropped me off at the old house. Gradually, my mind drifted back to the image of the tall handsome physician with the noble bearing and neatly combed gray hair, and I felt better, thinking maybe there was hope after all.

There was no hope. The tall physician with the gray hair could not save my father or the medical profession. My father's practice dwindled over the next five years, until he was forced to abandon his office altogether and sell its furnishings. Unable to work as a solo practitioner in the new managed care environment, he applied for full-time salaried positions but was unable to secure one despite his experience. His odd personality was likely a factor. After working here and there, he retired from medicine early, which depressed him, as he loved being a doctor. His back grew bent, as if a stone hung around his neck; he spent most of his time in a chair. It was sad to see this man, who for decades had stood ready at the drop of a hat to rush to a patient's aid, and whose very nature of life had accustomed him to continual movement, end his days of motion in the enforced sitting of retirement, marking time in one spot. He died in 2002 an unhappy man.

My mother suffered through the travails of being an ex-doctor's wife. "A dethroned queen," she called herself. No more party invitations came. Sometimes she would ask me to drive her past a doctor's house on an evening when a party was being held there. I would park the car on the street and let her stare at the house and listen to the laughter coming from inside and remember how it all once was. As I pulled away, a strange force would twist her neck and turn it back in the house's direction. The low point came at a wedding reception when she was forced to sit at a table in the back reserved for ex-doctors' wives. All the "rejects," she moaned pathetically. A kind of mini-leper colony. Fortunately, she was able to turn her misfortune into a career as a social worker, which she excelled at.

My grandfather's career as a physician began in failure and ended in success. My father's career began in success and ended in failure. The pivot around which both men's lives moved was the American ideal of the doctor. My grandfather could not adapt to that ideal. My father embraced it at the moment it began to unravel.

In the 1970s and 1980s, the physician ideal was attacked from every angle. As part scientist, the doctor was increasingly viewed as someone cold and heartless, and more interested in slotting patients into treatment categories than in listening to them. As part technician, the doctor was thought to be more interested in gadgetry than in people. Worse, gadgetry made medicine too expensive. Gadgetry was also something that non-MDs could master, making it easier for nurses and other health care professionals to challenge physician control. As part gentleman, the doctor was seen as protecting his monopoly against the intrusion of women and minorities into the profession. As part benefactor, well, doctors seemed to be as money-hungry as everyone else, and posing as benefactors simply made them look like hypocrites.

As the vision collapsed, professional medicine broke down again into competing schools, each declaiming on behalf of the scientist, the technician, the gentleman, or the benefactor. It was a rehash of the same fight American doctors had a century before. I watched this drama play out as a resident (described in this book's first chapter).

The story of my grandfather and father bears directly on the problem of medical catastrophes.

First, both my grandfather and my father were oddballs. Despite this, they were still able to practice medicine. In the new order, as doctors move from being independent practitioners to being dependent employees, on salary, they have less freedom to be oddballs. Oddball doctors sometimes even have difficulty finding good jobs. The system today prefers doctors who are good "company people," even though good company people do not necessarily make safe doctors.

Second, the politics of medicine were once quite interesting, even comical, because all the different players in medicine shared power. The doctors, the doctors' wives, the nurses, the Catholic sisters, the hospitals, and the insurance companies—each group had some power, but no group held all the power. Along with the silliness, real heartwarming social behavior flowed out of this way of life—for example, doctors sending expensive Christmas gifts every year to other doctors, or doctors giving the children of other doctors their first summer jobs. Some friendships were true; others were anchored in self-interest, an exchange of favors. But taken altogether, the silliness and the sweetness, the friendly gestures and the self-interested ones, humanized the practice of medicine.

Such charm and delicate sentiments waned when doctors became salaried employees. So did any feeling of independence. Immaculately dressed, clear-thinking businesspeople with all the facts before them took command. They spoke in geometric terms about human affairs, such as "the organizational processes affecting the annual case load," and so forth. They called doctors "providers." They threatened those providers with dismissal if they judged their performance to be inadequate. Health care itself became organized like a pyramid, with a corporate or hospital entity employing doctors and nurses, and enjoying the lion's share of power. While a pyramidal system is often successful administratively, it poses risks to patients clinically.

Third, both my father and my grandfather loved being doctors. To them, doctoring was more than just a job. It was an object of affection that they feared being torn away from. This attitude is less prevalent today. Many physicians now *do* think of doctoring as a job. This decreases the risk of medical catastrophes in some ways but in other ways raises it.

Each of these points will be discussed in the next three chapters.

7

WHEN DOCTORS LOSE CONTROL OF THEIR OWN PERSONALITIES

Early in my career, I knew an anesthesiologist named Dr. F. In his mid-fifties, originally from somewhere in the Caucasus, he was short, stout, and hairy, with a remarkable gift for making people feel warm and happy. His casual, free-and-easy way came not from any political conviction but from the simple fact that he liked people more than places, and places more than ideas. He found everyone interesting, listened attentively to their problems as if they were worthy of a memoir, and smiled sincerely. His only defect from the perspective of conventional morality was that he ogled pretty women. People knew how he was, but they gave him a pass, in part because he was so likeable but also because he was consistent; it was mostly change that caught people's attention and made them nervous. Had Dr. F once been a choirboy who started ogling women only recently, people would have complained. But his behavior was as it had always been. With his reputation established quick and early, and having been at the hospital for over twenty years, he and his antics were viewed as part of the normal backdrop of life.

One day, I walked into the operating room to give Dr. F a break. A young woman lay on the operating table half asleep, her strong muscular legs hanging in stirrups and slightly contracting against the force of gravity, her thin blue gown barely concealing her large bosom, which protruded upward and outward. The gynecologist, a short, weedy, bald man with a pencil neck, sat on a stool inches away from the patient's bottom, his head framed by the patient's legs, impatiently waiting to perform a D and C.

"Ah, young man, a break for me? You're a good fellow," Dr. F expounded, a broad smile tugging at the corners of his mask. "But first let me put the EKG leads on," he said, his eyes flickering sparks of lust.

"Is she asleep?" I asked him.

"Well, young man, that's a good question," he began, his large hairy hand moving across the woman's left breast, his fingers holding an EKG pad and looking like the talons of a giant prehistoric bird. Dr. F paused for a moment to concentrate, and then continued:

"Even when a woman is anesthetized, she'll protect herself down there, you know? Give her enough Pentothal to close her eyelids and she'll still snap her legs together faster than a clam in danger when touched. Give her some more Pentothal so that she barely breathes. Her legs drop nice and loose in the stirrups. You think you're all set, but watch and see, she'll knock those legs together the instant she's touched. Give her some more Pentothal. Make her stop breathing altogether. Why, she still shuts her legs—even when she's turning blue! She'll die before opening those legs. Lord in Heaven! You've got to inject enough Pentothal to drop her blood pressure before she'll surrender her honor. Amazing, isn't it? I call it God's protective reflex. He gave it to all women, even the ugly ones—the Lord is just—to prevent men from taking advantage of them. It's wisdom for life, my boy."

While Dr. F lectured, the gynecologist applied a sharp instrument to the patient's bottom without telling anyone. Suddenly the woman's heart rate jumped. Before Dr. F or I could react, the woman, although unconscious, wrapped her legs around the surgeon's neck and squeezed. Unable to free himself, he cried for help. The operating room nurse tried to pry the woman's legs apart but failed. Things grew serious as the women's strong legs threatened to twist the surgeon's head off its pedicle or choke off his air supply. Almost by instinct Dr. F injected a slug of Pentothal into the woman's intravenous. Within ten seconds her legs relaxed and the gynecologist escaped.

"Damn you, F!" cried the gynecologist.

"My boy, there you are! Just as I told you!" Dr. F joked, patting me on the back. The nurse retreated to the back of the room, convulsing with silent laughter.

The gynecologist shook his head to check for injury and then dove back into work, too embarrassed to look around the room.

That was Dr. F.

The next day, a drug rep served lunch for the anesthesia department. Everyone knew it would be a good meal, as catered lunches were once a way for drug companies to entice doctors to use their products. There was noticeable animation in the lounge when the rep walked in with four hot trays wrapped in tin foil. People nimbly jockeyed for position around the crowded table.

Dr. F ate three helpings. Afterward, fuddled by his heavy meal, he quietly smiled. He had worked the previous night, and before lunch his fatigue had been painfully apparent. Shakily had he made his way to the lounge to eat, stumbling toward the door, moving in little spurts, as if fighting a heavy wind. Now he sat contentedly in his chair, refreshed and cheerful. A post-call doctor needs so little. He has only to get a bit farther away from death and disease as usual, sit in a comfortable chair, eat a good meal, and up it comes, the fast-ripening doctor's happiness.

Dr. F's next patient was waiting for him in the holding area. When he rose to his feet he looked weary again, but joyfully so, almost giddy. He wandered over to see his patient, a massively obese woman scheduled for weight-reduction surgery. His bloodshot eyes looked a bit crazed as he interviewed her. I listened in while waiting for my own patient to arrive.

"I've tried so hard to lose weight," the woman wept halfway through the interview.

"I know, dear, I know," Dr. F cosseted her without restraint, putting his hairy hand on her arm and stroking it. "But after the surgery, you'll look wonderful. You have such a lovely face. Why, when I saw you from a distance I thought, 'I don't know what her name is, but she's not just a woman, she's beauty itself!'" he said with conviction, although his speech was slightly drunken-sounding.

"Really?" she replied, somewhat embarrassed.

"Now there's no reason to be modest," Dr. F went on delightedly, his wide smile crinkling the dark circles under his eyes. "Why, you're like whipped butter! In a few months every man will be trying to spread you on slices of bread and eat them."

"But I'll still be big," she moaned.

"Not big. Strong! That's very attractive. Why, when I was a young man I dated a first-class wrestler, in the top grade. Now, I was strong, too, in those days. It was before I became a doctor. I could carry a rug on each shoulder anywhere I liked, but even so this woman would get around me, just above the knee, and by the shoulder, and she would flip me over and pin me to the mattress. Oh, what a woman! Don't worry. It was all done with love. And if it hadn't been for the war, I would have sat happily on a branch with her for the rest of my life. We would have been like love birds. But she found a young lieutenant . . ."

A nurse interrupted their conversation and told them it was time to go back to the operating room.

Whistling softly to himself, Dr. F helped wheel the woman back to the operating room and within five minutes had her asleep. With fatigue creeping back over him, and so much food in his stomach, he grew sleepy himself. Feeling cold he went out into the hall to get two blankets from the warmer. He wrapped one around his shoulders and the second around his waist. Then he nodded off. Toward the end of the case, he woke up and rushed to catch up on his charting. Absent-mindedly, thinking of other things, he injected morphine into the intravenous—a drug the patient had a known allergy to. Within minutes the woman turned beet red, her blood pressure dropped, and her lungs tightened. Dr. F grew startled and called for help, but by the time I and another doctor had rushed in, he had injected adrenalin and remedied the situation.

In the recovery room the woman asked Dr. F why she was so red.

"I'm afraid you had an allergic reaction to the morphine," he replied sheepishly.

"Oh, I'm so sorry!" she countered. "I think I told you about that. I'm allergic to morphine. I hope I didn't cause you too much trouble. I'm so sorry!"

Dr. F patted her hand and told her there was no need to apologize. Afterward I whispered to him, "You give her a drug she's allergic to and *she's* the one who apologizes?" Dr. F winked playfully and said nothing.

On one level, this story says something obvious about catastrophe prevention: tired doctors are more likely to cause catastrophes than well-rested ones are, especially in anesthesiology. Dr. F should have gone home that morning and not put that patient to sleep. Yet this story also says something important about doctor-patient relationships, and what it means to be a doctor.

Patients will often accept a few mistakes from their doctors if their doctors befriend them, as Dr. F befriended his. That's because there's nothing more painful than ending a friendship. An injured patient eagerly sues his doctor if his doctor treats him like an insignificant nothing. He gets to turn the tables and treat his doctor with even greater contempt than he was treated. But when a doctor and a patient are friends, the patient often wants to forget about his doctor's mistakes and pretend that they never happened. Because if they did happen, and the patient sues his doctor, then he'll have to call his doctor something other than "friend," and nothing is more painful than breaking with a friend. Lawyers will advise the patient to reconsider, but he won't. The patient feels his doctor is his own kind, a kindred spirit. "Yes, you're right," the patient will tell his lawyer. "I'm injured. But that's just one side of my life . . . what you don't see . . . there are *other reasons*." And the patient forgives.

Yet being friends is not the same as being equals. This is a mistake that doctors often make, especially today, as patients have more access to medical information, thereby narrowing the gap between what doctors and patients know, while the health care system turns patients into consumers, or even colleagues, with both doctor and patient "working together" to fight disease. Lawsuits are more likely in this environment. As doctors try in every way to be democratic and treat their patients like respected colleagues, patients almost start to imagine themselves real doctors, with medical opinions that deserve to be taken seriously. When a doctor sees this happening, his or her democratic instinct is to think, "Okay, I'm not proud. I don't mind if my patient thinks he and I are on the same level. We'll both be doctors." But later, if injured, the patient, who now imagines himself on a par with real doctors, thinks scornfully of his doctor, that he (the patient) earned the title of doctor by reading a few websites, while the doctor went to medical school and yet, despite his extra education, still made a mistake. The patient sues almost on principle, to rid his profession of hacks.

Dr. F often befriended his patients, but he never treated them as equals. At the same time, he never allowed his friendship with patients to cross over into true intimacy, in part because it was unprofessional, but also because it would have kept him from reacting properly during a crisis. Dr. F's relationship with patients existed in its own space: he was both a friend and a master to his patients.

When patients go to doctors, they entrust the directing of their health to professionals whose minds they regard as more powerful than their own. Some patients are more deferential than others, and some patients argue more than others, but all patients possess a master in their doctor. They never cease to draw on doctors' minds, and they do so with a prejudice in their doctor's favor. Yet patients also have a friend in their doctor. That doesn't mean patients and doctors agree on all subjects. Sometimes they may disagree entirely on important issues—as friends do. But doctors and patients do share the same hopes and face the same disappointments. What doctors and patients enjoy is friendship on a high level, one that is free of jealousy because they share a common objective. The doctor works hard for the patient. The patient, in turn, works hard at getting better. Satisfaction prevails because both are busy and there is little time for ill feelings to develop. And yet, despite their friendship, the patient still recognizes the doctor as the moving spirit in the relationship.

For this dynamic to work, doctors must accept patients as they are in the same way that friends accept their friends in everyday life. This is why doctors must be more artists than craftspeople. Doctors and patients do not live together, and therefore doctors lack the opportunity to appraise their patients the way prospective friends appraise each other every day at the school lunch table or at the officers' mess hall. Doctors must innovate to compensate for the lack of time they spend with patients. Sometimes doctors must apply the methods of the philosopher and the novelist to understand their patients en route to accepting them.

But patients must also accept their doctors. This is why Dr. F's oddball personality worked so well. A doctor's intelligence and scientific accuracy will not always gain his or her patient's acceptance. On the contrary, many patients fear the opinion of a mind that is too lucid. They prefer to be friends with someone less exacting. They prefer in their doctors a few amiable weaknesses added to the high qualities. There is something inhuman in absolute perfection that overwhelms the mind and heart; it may command respect, but it keeps friendship at a distance through discouragement and humiliation. Patients are often glad when a great doctor reassures them of his or her humanity by possessing a few peculiarities. And peculiarities Dr. F had aplenty.

So did my father and grandfather. Both men were oddballs. My grandfather's weirdness hobbled him in private practice because he was weird in a way that many patients disliked. That doesn't devalue the importance of weirdness in doctors. Eventually my grandfather found an audience that did appreciate him, at the Old Soldiers' Home. He liked the old soldiers and they liked him. As for my father, his patients warmed to his brand of weirdness. I hated his corny jokes, but his patients liked them. He once asked me in front of a patient if I was "corn-fused" (a play on "confused"). I thought the play on words stupid, but his patient laughed and laughed.

Friendship works through a hidden fraternity of spirit; the act of friendship itself is an obscure ordering in which it is impossible to find a rule or law. This is why tutorials on the doctor-patient relationship are useless, or worse, downright irritating. They try to transform the miracle of friendship into an algorithm, to turn sentiment into a program, to anchor the doctor-patient relationship in "effective methods" and "achievable measurable goals." Better to let doctors just be themselves and for patients to select them on the basis of idiosyncrasies that harmonize with their own. It is why patients hate it when insurance companies restrict what doctors they can go to. It's not just that patients fear getting a lousy doctor; it's also that they fear getting a doctor whom they are not in sync with, and who is not weird in the same way they are.

I watched carefully how Dr. F put patients at ease.

One day, while on obstetrics, he helped me get a patient ready for a cesarean section. The woman was obese, which can complicate placement of a spinal anesthetic. I methodically cleaned the woman's back with alcohol, sweeping the series of drenched swabs over her skin in ever widening circles. The woman bent her fat waist in a bow. Syringe in hand, I warned her from behind that a small needle stick was coming. "You're going to feel a little prick," I said.

Dr. F, who was facing the woman on the other side, whispered to her, "A little prick? That's how you got into this mess. Right?" He chuckled. The woman outright laughed, her fat back jiggling with emotion. I passed the larger spinal needle. No cerebrospinal fluid returned. I passed the needle again and again, but there was no spinal space, no bone, no noth-

ing. Dr. F distracted her with more lewd humor. The woman giggled with
each joke, giving me more time to poke around and find the right spot. A
few minutes later, I found it and injected the anesthetic.

We rolled the woman on her back. The nurses prepped her abdomen.
Despite our warnings, the woman kept reaching for her abdomen, threatening the field's sterility. In all her nervous excitement about having a
baby, she kept forgetting to keep still. By now her husband was sitting
next to her; yet he had no more luck in calming her down than we did.
Finally we taped her arms down against the armboards to keep them from
moving. Because the woman was scared, and slightly claustrophobic, Dr.
F defused the situation with a shameless tease. "Don't worry, I'm just
tying you down so you don't reach over and pinch the surgeon's butt," he
said. He laughed, while the woman and her husband laughed along with
him. The rest of the surgery was uneventful.

I decided to use Dr. F's line in the future. And I needed "a good line."
I wasn't very good at putting people at ease. Many young doctors lack
this social skill. When they go to a party or meet new people for dinner,
they know that if they talk about their important medical cases or enlarge
on their own decisions that vitally affected a case, people will listen with
rapt attention. They don't need the social graces to converse, and so those
graces remain underdeveloped. Many young doctors rationalize away
their limitations, thinking that at least people can learn things from them,
compared to everyday banter, where people are left bored after speaking
with someone who talks about everything but only lightly touches on
anything, and people get nothing out of it. Talk with a doctor at least
leaves a person edified, they think. But when caring for patients, a doctor
really does have to be able to charm patients, to put them at ease. That's
why I wanted "a line."

Three days later, I was managing another cesarian section on obstetrics. My patient was nervous and reaching for her abdomen, as my earlier
patient had. I taped her arms to the armboards and, with her husband
present, frenetically uttered Dr. F's line about not wanting her to reach
over and pinch the surgeon's butt. There was gaiety in my tone. I chuckled after my delivery and said nothing more so the couple would know it
was the punch line.

I expected laughter. Instead, there was dead silence. The patient stiff-
ened and turned her face away, while afterward her husband complained
that I had been flirting with his wife.

What went wrong?

On one level I had been a bad actor. Sometimes medical practice is a large stage on which an endless play is going on. Doctors must connect with their patients in the same way that actors must connect with their audience. Sometimes actors cannot connect in their roles simply because of who they are. Dr. F was old and wrinkled, whereas I was young and succulent; at my age, I should have never used that line with a female patient. Yet actors can also be bad, especially if they try to connect in a forcible way as I had. My "line" obviously had a studied, bookish flavor. I had defeated my own object, as the forced friendliness destroyed the illusion of friendship the line was intended to create.

Yet the deeper problem was that I *had* been acting. Dr. F had not. When Dr. F had uttered the line, he had simply been himself. Instead of thinking, "This is what a doctor who wants to be my friend says," his patient probably thought, "A friend is saying this." Dr. F was an oddball. Nevertheless, he was authentic. The feeling of friendship patients experienced with him was also authentic. It's why patients liked him.

The following week I was on the obstetrics ward again. An overhead call announced an emergency cesarian section. I rushed into the operating room. The patient was a young Japanese woman who spoke no English. She was lying on the operating room table and shivering in fear. No translators were immediately available in those days, and so it was impossible for me to take a quick medical history. The only thing the obstetrician could tell me was that the woman had a history of angioedema. In that disease people swell in different parts of their bodies, including in their airways, in response to an allergen. The airway swelling can be severe enough to cause suffocation.

"What do you mean by 'angioedema'?" I asked him with concern while checking my anesthesia equipment.

"Just what I said. She has a history of angioedema," the obstetrician replied matter-of-factly, thinking the information not especially important. "Now put her down. I need to get the baby out."

"Yes, but there are different kinds of angioedema. What kind is hers?" I asked, rushing to place monitors on the patient.

"Hell, I don't know. Maybe she swells when she eats sushi," the obstetrician teased. "Now get going."

"Fine, but why would you even know that? Do you ask every patient if she swells when she eats sushi?" I asked, connecting my syringes to the patient's intravenous and preparing to inject.

"Listen, she's had angioedema all her life. That's all I know. I don't remember how I know. Maybe her husband told me. I guess they start eating sushi pretty early over there," the obstetrician joked. Then, growing more serious, he barked, "Now let's go!"

"Hereditary angioedema"—the phrase raced through my mind. She might have that particular variant of the disease if it had been a problem all her life. It is the most dangerous kind. Not just allergens trigger swelling; simple instrumentation can also cause it—for example, putting a laryngoscope in a patient's mouth when inducing general anesthesia. Nor can the swelling be treated with epinephrine, unlike other allergic reactions. The disease involves a blood protein deficiency. Airway swelling must be treated with fresh frozen plasma.

I hesitated for a moment, then decided to forego general anesthesia—to avoid airway instrumentation—and place a quick spinal anesthetic. The small delay put the baby at risk, but my first duty was to the mother. Also, the patient was thin; I felt confident I could get a spinal in her in less than a minute.

I asked the nurses to help me flip the woman onto her side so I could get to her back. The obstetrician protested and called me "ridiculous," but I ignored him. I tore open the spinal set, cleaned the patient's back, inserted the spinal needle, found the right spot on the first pass, and injected the anesthetic—all in less than a minute. Because it was an emergency I used lidocaine, a drug with short duration but quick onset. The obstetrician cut. A healthy baby emerged from the patient's abdomen one minute later.

We were home free. Then the obstetrician ran into some bleeding that kept the case from finishing. Thirty minutes later, the patient moaned in pain. Since lidocaine should last forty minutes, I decided anxiety was probably exacerbating her pain, and that she still had some anesthesia left. The obstetrician said he needed twenty more minutes. I gave the woman some intravenous sedation to calm her down, but there was a limit to how much I could give her. She had eaten a full meal two hours before. If she went to sleep without a breathing tube in place, she might vomit and aspirate her stomach contents, which could kill her. To go to sleep, she would require an endotracheal tube—but that risked a bout of angioedema.

Her moaning grew worse. In the most stupid American way, I tried telling her that we would only be ten more minutes. I spoke English slowly. I spoke English loudly. It had no effect. She cried and screamed. I reached for the Pentothal and muscle relaxant and prepared to induce general anesthesia.

Suddenly, Dr. F walked in. I informed him of the situation. I asked him to inject the drugs so I could intubate. He motioned me to put the drugs away. Then he took off his mask and stared directly into the patient's eyes. He spoke words that I did not understand.

"*Kam hitch um hot ho!*" he said to her, harshly, as if giving her an order.

The woman quieted down and stared back at him.

"*Uh-h-h do kee ha ai-raku!*" Dr. F declared forcefully.

Transfixed, the woman kept staring at Dr. F. Then she quietly replied, "*Ah so.*"

Dr. F continued. "*Ne ha so tu,*" he said. In a tone that made him sound very wise, he followed up with "*Des ka nu so ha.*"

The woman kept staring at Dr. F, her eyes sparkling with amazement. "*Ah so,*" she said again.

Their dialogue continued for several more minutes, with the woman replying "*Ah so*" each time. She was now quiet and calm.

The obstetrician raced to finish the surgery. He placed the last suture ten minutes later. As the drapes came down, both he and I thanked Dr. F profusely for his help.

I went to visit the patient during my postoperative rounds the following day. A translator was present. I asked her if she remembered me. Through the translator she said, "Yes." I asked her if she had any after-effects from the spinal anesthetic. She said, "No."

Then she asked me, "Who was that funny man in the operating room?"

"The man speaking with you? That was Dr. F," I replied.

"He was a funny man. He spoke words I didn't understand," she said.

"What?" I said, a little startled. "He was speaking to you in Japanese, wasn't he?"

The woman continued, "He must have been speaking a foreign language. But I felt I could understand him. I thought he was telling me that I was all right, and that everything would be all right."

Speechless, I simply nodded my head and left.

I saw Dr. F later that day. I told him what the woman had said.

"You weren't speaking Japanese to her, were you?" I asked him.

Dr. F smiled and said nothing.

"You don't speak Japanese, do you?" I asked, desperate for some kind of explanation.

Still smiling, he patted me on the shoulder, winked playfully, and walked on.

His weirdness had averted a potential catastrophe.

Life pushed Dr. F and me onto separate paths. Years later, I heard about the troubles he had toward the end of his career when he became an employed physician.

The first salvo came when he told a nurse who had changed her hairstyle that she looked "sexy." The nurse, who was angry with Dr. F for other reasons, complained. The company chastised Dr. F, who was truly confused, as he thought he was paying the woman a compliment. The company told him to behave. But now Dr. F was unsure what it meant to behave. Unfamiliar with the new rules governing corporate America, he was like a man who moves around without the use of his senses, beset by traps. He talked less at work. He also avoided social events, such as Christmas parties, as these were now considered extensions of the workplace, making them sources of risk.

Although Dr. F self-censored, his unique style nevertheless peeped through. One day, a technician asked him over the phone to silence a beep on an anesthesia machine. Dr. F was busy at the time, so he told the technician to press a certain button. The technician told Dr. F that he had to do it. Harried, but still in good humor, Dr. F replied, "Okay, but you know, it's not rocket science." The technician complained, accusing Dr. F of fostering a "hostile work environment." On another occasion, a nurse put a small intravenous in a patient going for surgery that would potentially have high blood loss. When Dr. F saw it he humorously corrected the nurse with the patient nearby, saying, "You couldn't suck enough water through that straw to survive in the desert." While Dr. F placed a larger intravenous, the nurse complained to Dr. F's superior, saying Dr. F shouldn't have corrected her in front of the patient. The complaint made its way up through the ranks of officialdom. Again, Dr. F found himself in trouble. In the end, he decided to retire early. The company was happy to see him go.

Doctors reading this book may laugh at Dr. F. Part of me laughs at Dr. F. But such laughter is a sad indication of what doctors have become. Doctors laugh because they know that in order to avoid trouble these days one has to be exquisitely sensitive to other people's feelings. No careless quips. If one is foolish enough to be weird, one should at least take good care not to display that weirdness in front of others. The smart person today follows the rules and displays outward obedience to them, even if he or she has nothing but contempt for them. The main thing is order and system. Now is not the time of the weird people. It is the time of the flexible people, the people who know how to bend at the right moment. It is the time of the company people who shave off their idiosyncrasies to fit in and belong. That's how a doctor today avoids trouble. From that perspective, Dr. F was a fool.

My parents trained me to be a company man. They instilled in me mental radar that let me discern what other people were thinking so that I could tailor my behavior accordingly. As a child, whenever I asked my mother what I should do in a particular situation, she would invariably reply, "Well, what are all the other kids doing?" In solid 1950s fashion I learned the importance of being liked and fitting in. Later, when I became a doctor, I decided this education had been unnecessary, since doctors, unlike company men, had the freedom to be themselves, including the freedom to be weird. But as doctors increasingly become employees, that education has proved valuable after all.

The problem for patients is that good company people do not necessarily make good doctors. They do not necessarily prevent catastrophes. A doctor's weirdness has nothing to do with his or her ability to practice medicine well.

I have known several outstanding doctors in my career who were oddballs.

I knew a German-born anesthesiologist who specialized in putting children to sleep. Built like a medium-sized bear, he would sit children on his lap to anesthetize them, while his muscular legs would squeeze their spindly legs to prevent them from kicking. High-minded and stubborn, distrustful of others, angry at the world, and without an ounce of coziness, he took his woes and burdens with him wherever he went. Few people liked him; many children feared him. "Do you have any bra-thers?" he would ask a child in a thick German accent, his painful way of trying to be pleasant. "Do you like spa-ghet-ti?" he would ask in a guttural tone. Sometimes the child would wail and struggle, prompting him to tighten his hold on the child and declare, "*Ach*, you little brat!" Yet he was an outstanding doctor. He saved lives.

I knew an anesthesiologist from Latin America with a bad temper. He would flare up like gunpowder in the face of any patronizing reference to his origins and rarely controlled himself in time. Most of his anger was real, although some of it was slightly calculated, like a dog's snarl, a way of telling an offender not to go there or to leave things alone. Once begun, his tantrums stopped only when they ran out of fuel; he yelled, he berated, and on one occasion he put his fist through a wall and broke a bone. Curiously, despite the habit of distrust and constant vigilance that had insinuated itself into his personality, he was at heart a kind individual. Watching children suffer especially pained him. He was a complex character. He was also an outstanding doctor. He saved lives.

I knew an anesthesiologist from the Midwest. Straight-laced and reserved, he had the aura of the scoutmaster about him. He was incredibly thorough during his patient intakes. Sometimes he would interview healthy patients for almost an hour before giving them anesthesia, probing for a history of even minor ailments, such as sexually transmitted diseases, looking at patients with parental severity, speaking to them in icy tones, and driving some of them crazy. But even at his most distant, he was engrossed in his patients, studying them with all-knowing eyes, while to his colleagues he was cold and sober beyond need simply because he was complete and didn't require their society. He didn't spend time thinking about what other people thought of him. Yet he was an outstanding doctor. He saved lives.

These anesthesiologists would have difficulty finding employment today. There are few institutional laws that I can point to as the reason for their difficulty; it all belongs in the category of unwritten laws of behavior. Their personalities would make them socially undesirable. They would make bad company people. Nevertheless, they were good doctors.

Many American doctors today are good company people. They all come from the same incubator; they're marked with different-colored inks, but there's essentially no difference. Their behavior is in exact conformity with existing prescriptions. No rough edges. At work they talk like NPR; their words rarely contain a single living emotion. At best, they are people who avoid revealing the whole of their thought; they are different from how they are in real life; they are a people constrained and held in check. Other doctors are company people to their very bones. They say what is expected of them; they are inconspicuous; they weigh their words carefully even while joking; they know the importance of being politically correct; they will never start revolutions; they will never hurl challenges or level accusations against their bosses; they are easy to move with carrots and sticks; they are easy to intimidate with threats to their employment. Because they are paid well they are simultaneously self-satisfied and scared. In sum, they are completely harmless people.

Corporate America is not to blame for the rise of the company culture in medicine. Corporate America is what it is. Since the 1950s, it has preferred to employ company people. The result has been great success. From cars to toothpaste, corporate America produces vital products at low cost. Yet taking care of patients is different from making cars or toothpaste. More risk is involved, and the company personality is not only irrelevant to the defraying of that risk but also a distraction from the core elements needed to do so.

The medical profession is to blame for the rise of the company culture in medicine. That culture filled a void that opened up when the medical profession no longer knew what a doctor should be.

First, the doctor-as-technician model that replaced the old vision of what a doctor should be enabled the corporate takeover of medicine. Before, when doctoring involved a complex set of qualities and attributes, and not just technical wizardry, the notion that business executives could "manage" doctors using fixed rules and procedures would have been inconceivable. It would have been like telling ministers to sermonize with one or two words, or telling painters to paint with one or two colors. Doctoring, like preaching and painting, was not merely a craft but also an art that required a broad grasp of humanity and subtle intelligence. But technicians are easy to manage. Their tools are predictable. Their thinking is predictable. Their output is predictable. Business executives like to manage workers whose decision trees follow a few simple pathways.

When doctors became technicians they paved the way for business executives to come in and manage them, too.

Second, medical schools began to select for company people among their applicants. This represents a significant change from the past.

In the 1930s and 1940s, when the company culture cemented itself in American corporate life, prospective job applicants took personality tests to show they were loyal, well-adjusted, able to get along with people, and politically correct (which in those days meant conservative). During this same period, medical schools focused almost exclusively on their applicants' scientific aptitude. No personality tests were used to screen future doctors. In the 1950s, medical schools encouraged applicants to take classes in the humanities; yet this wasn't personality screening so much as a cue to applicants to be both good scientists and well-rounded gentlemen. In the 1960s, as the technology race between the United States and the former Soviet Union heated up, medical schools reemphasized scientific aptitude. Indeed, many prospective medical students during this period applied with the intention of being biomechanical engineers.[1] An applicant's personality went largely unknown.

During the 1990s, in the name of "professionalism," medical schools began to screen for student attitudes.[2] This was not yet the company culture. On the contrary, the purpose of such screening was not to graduate company people but to avoid doing so. Medical schools feared doctors working under managed care might be more loyal to the companies they worked for than to their patients. Classes were held to teach students to put patients first.

But the door was opened for more behavioral modeling. In 2005, the American Medical Association pushed a new initiative to give a medical school applicant's personality more weight in the selection process. Physicians had a sense that a doctor should be more than just a scientist or a technician, but they weren't quite sure what a doctor should be. They settled on an applicant with excellent social radar, someone who excelled in getting along with others, who worked well within an organization, and who embraced popular cultural values. They wanted an applicant who would pay close attention to the signals he or she received from others, and who would adjust his or her behavior accordingly; a person who would be liked by others, and who would want and need to be liked; a person who would seek the approval of his or her peers, and who, when getting that approval, would desire more approval; a person who would be at home anywhere and nowhere, and who was capable of a superficial intimacy with everyone. In other words, they wanted an applicant with a certain personality—the same personality sought by American companies in the 1950s.[3]

In 2010, the American Association of Medical Colleges joined the initiative, publishing a grab bag of virtues, such as compassion, the ability to function as part of a team, dependability, adaptability, altruism, high enthusiasm, and conscientiousness—again, the same traits that companies screened potential employees for in the 1950s.[4] More than half of U.S. medical schools now screen for one or more personality traits among their applicants.[5] The medical school entrance exam (or MCAT) was also adjusted to screen for the company personality. The personality exams of the 1950s screened for conservative tendencies; today's MCAT screens for liberal ones, such as tolerance and political sensitivity, but the principle is the same.[6]

Medical schools push the company personality in a second way. Their list of desirable personality traits is long and almost impossible to find in one person. Medical schools want a rose without thorns, an angel without wings. They want a perfect creature. Instead, they get people who know how to transcend an application and give examiners what they are looking for; they get people who know how to *appear* as perfect creatures. In the 1950s, journalist William Whyte described such people in *The Organization Man*. Referring to applicants to corporate training programs, he wrote, "They are predisposed to read a good bit more between the lines than many of their elders would like them to."[7] In medicine today, these people exist among the thousands of applicants who pay premed consulting companies to help them write the perfect essay to convey all the desired personality traits.

Sadly, a good company person does not necessarily make a good doctor. Good company people excel at using the system to protect themselves. When a catastrophe occurs, they know the importance in company warfare of thinking quicker than others, and of getting your blow in first, before the bureaucracy starts to crank. They know how to show how seemingly unconnected incidents in their lives fit into a pattern, which, taken as a whole, is exonerating. They know how an affable personality works as vital social capital to draw upon when one's medical abilities are suddenly called into question. They know all these things because they excel at knowing what their supervisors are looking for. After all, they started their medical careers by writing a personal statement about why they wanted to be a doctor, thinking the whole time about the admissions officer who would read that statement, check it against their attached autobiography, compare one answer with another, comb for contradictions, and put a plus or minus after each sentence. They knew the application was a game, just as they know that saving their skins is a game. They know how to play both games. But they do not necessarily know how to rescue a patient from a catastrophe.

Here is one example: To maximize efficiency and worker productivity, many hospitals today want their operating rooms to start simultaneously. If a hospital start time is, say, 7:45 AM, then a mad rush occurs at 7:43 AM. Employed doctors and nurses desperately push to get their patient into their particular operating room to avoid being penalized. Indeed, if they have too many late starts on their record, they risk being fired. Already at 7:44 AM, the surgeon, the anesthesiologist, the nurse, and the orderly—all company employees—are plotting how to offload blame for a potential late start onto someone else.

In one hospital on the West Coast, an anesthesiologist interviewed his patient at 7:20 AM. He thought his patient, who had recently experienced some mild chest pain, needed more cardiac workup, including a second EKG, which would push the operating room start time well past 7:45 AM. He looked on the sheet the hospital gave to doctors and nurses to justify a late start. There were boxes to be checked if the late start was the anesthesiologist's fault, the surgeon's fault, or the nurse's fault; there was a box for when the patient arrived late at the hospital; there was also a box for a delay in getting the patient's lab results. But there was no box for when a second EKG was needed. The anesthesiologist panicked. He knew that if he delayed the case to perform the second EKG, then his box, the anesthesiologist's box, would get checked and he would be blamed. He had already been associated with several other late starts. Those late starts had not been his fault; nevertheless, administrators were watching—they had told him they were watching. He decided to forego the second EKG and bring the patient in at 7:45 AM.

During surgery the patient suffered a myocardial infarction and almost died. Afterward, the anesthesiologist tried to weasel out of all blame. He told the administrators that the need for the second EKG had been questionable. He downplayed the patient's chest pain that had spurred him to seek the second EKG. He gave a thoughtful explanation about how medicine is an inexact science. He was proactive and asked to be on a committee that would review similar situations going forward. He talked about formulating new policies. He advocated for more input from nursing and other departments. He discussed reaching out. The administrators loved it. He spoke their language, which reassured them; he shared in their ideas fully. True, they probably knew he was afraid of losing his job; yet they also knew that fear is what made the 7:45 AM policy work. A scared anesthesiologist is an efficient anesthesiologist. So they let him off.

I would rather be taken care of by an oddball.

Medical schools may argue that graduating doctors need a company personality to secure employment in the emerging health care order. Yet it is not the medical schools' job to do corporate medicine's bidding. Their job is to produce the best and safest doctors they can, even if that means graduating oddballs. To prevent catastrophes, it is corporate medicine that must adjust, not the medical training programs.

8

WHEN DOCTORS LOSE CONTROL OF THEIR OWN RULES

Ms. O was a morbidly obese sixty-year-old woman with a history of reflux and severe asthma needing an emergency hip pinning. In the back of my mind, I had already decided on spinal anesthesia, since general anesthesia with a breathing tube risked an asthma attack. But while reviewing Ms. O's labs I noticed that her platelet count was seventy-seven thousand, which was low, putting her at increased risk of bleeding. Bleeding at the operative site wasn't the problem so much as bleeding around her spine from the spinal needle. This rare but dreaded complication, called an *epidural hematoma*, can put pressure on the spinal cord and even cause paralysis. In the past, the rule among anesthesiologists was that at least a hundred thousand platelets were needed to safely place a spinal needle. Later studies dropped that number to eighty thousand, especially if the doctor had good reason to place a spinal—as, for example, in a patient with severe asthma. A few doctors will insert spinal needles in patients with fewer than eighty thousand platelets, as the risk of epidural hematoma increases arithmetically as one drops below eighty thousand, such that a patient with seventy-seven thousand platelets has only slightly more risk than a patient with eighty thousand platelets. Below fifty thousand platelets no anesthesiologist will go.

I was in a quandary. I really wanted to use spinal anesthesia, but the number "77,000" kept staring me in the face. Yes, it was below the magic "80,000"; then again, maybe the patient's real number was 80,000, and the difference was merely lab error. Even then, 77,000 was close to 80,000.

I must have looked doubtful, as Ms. O asked me, "Is everything all right, doctor?" Rather than confess the truth, I feigned nonchalance and said, "Everything is fine." Why did I hesitate to tell her my concerns at that moment? Because I saw myself as a scientist, and a scientist hates to admit ignorance of anything. A scientist thinks himself disgraced if he has to reply, "I'm not sure."

My father was less anxious about being caught without an answer. If a patient asked him a hard question, my father would often put the tip of his reading glasses in his mouth, ponder the question in silence for several seconds, and say, "I don't know," or "We shall see." Doing so never embarrassed him. He readily accepted the notion that doctors cannot have an answer for everything and must often choose a course with some doubt. To change his views, to admit to the change, and to appear changeable was the "gentleman" side to being a doctor, he once told me, compared to the scientific side, where precise laws determine a course of action.

Many doctors today feel vulnerable when they have no ready answer to give patients. It makes them feel like bad doctors. It also unnerves them to have to think individually and to choose a course without the security of a defined rule to back them up. They hate vagueness. When learning about a new drug, for example, they will wait for the drug rep to tell them the drug's loading dose, the dose frequency, the side effects, and the cost. They want to know figures and advantages, expressed in numbers. There is security in numbers. Other gadgets are sold to them in similar manner. Nothing abstract. No philosophy. The doctors are told the numbers. These are the figures. That is understandable. The doctors are happy with that. The pattern is repeated when they learn new approaches to disease management. They eagerly await the last slide at a conference when everything is summed up in the form of a therapeutic algorithm: if the number is this, then do this; if the number is that, then do that. Although patients resent being crammed into a treatment algorithm, they overlook the peace of mind that many doctors enjoy when they know what to do, at all times and in all cases, based on an algorithm.

I showed another anesthesiologist Ms. O's lab report. When she saw the number "77,000," she froze. The hypnosis of simple figures can act with remarkable power on doctors. She knew why I wanted to do the spinal, but she was also aware of the "eighty thousand platelet rule." She gave me very circumspect and enigmatic advice. "I suppose I would consider doing a spinal. It's a reasonable thing to consider," she said.

I reread the platelet studies, but moved no closer to a decision. I began to think that some paradox was hidden in the "eighty thousand platelet" rule. When pondering something intangible, as, for example, the idea of justice or virtue, the worm of self-doubt naturally crawls into my mind, and I cannot help asking myself, "Does this mean the same thing to everybody?" A scientific rule, in contrast, is supposed to mean the same thing to everyone. And yet the platelet rule could be interpreted in different ways and mean different things to different people. This made the rule useless, even dangerous, for a doctor never knows for sure how much individual judgment to use when working with a vague rule. The rule becomes like a map whose contours are confused and whose boundaries keep shifting; nevertheless one feels obligated to use the map constantly. A vague rule can befog doctors and make them act counter to their own consciences.

I asked another colleague. He winced when I gave him the patient's history. "I guess you're screwed either way," he said, referring to the inevitable malpractice suit. Ms. O's platelet count was destined to usher in a new chapter in my life, it seemed. A glimpse of beggarly destitution, after my trial, flashed through my head.

I asked a third anesthesiologist. He declared, "No way! Don't do a spinal!" I was inclined to agree with him; yet I could see that his instinct for self-preservation had been aroused, and I wondered how much it was affecting the integrity of his thought processes. A doctor thinks with his mind. A doctor also thinks with his body, as when placing an intravenous or a breathing tube. But sometimes, like an animal, a doctor thinks with the herd. If panic seizes a flock of sheep, each animal runs with the flock, not because it understands the reason for the panic but because it has an instinct that teaches the sheep that if it does not follow the flock, it will be at the mercy of its enemies. My colleague seemed to be thinking with the herd and hewing closely to the platelet rule to stay out of danger.

As I thought further about what to do, a nurse anesthetist approached me and asked me what I was doing. I told him I was trying to decide whether to put a spinal in a patient with seventy-seven thousand platelets. The nurse anesthetist haughtily replied, "Maybe you didn't know this, but eighty thousand is the limit." I shot back, "I know the rule." The nurse anesthetist snickered, "Some doctors don't. And if you didn't, now you do. Because I told you." I could see how his mind was working. The more rules he knew, the more on par with doctors he felt himself to be, for, to his mind, what makes a doctor is knowing the rules, just as, to his mind, what makes a doctor is knowing how to do procedures.

In the end I asked the most senior anesthesiologist in the department. "I wish I could tell you the right course," she responded. "But I can't. I think you're probably okay if you do a spinal, but I can't say for sure."

"So I'll be okay, until the point when I'm not okay," I replied.

"I'm afraid so," she said, sheepishly.

Such was her advice and warning: Follow medicine's rules, but sometimes don't follow them; sometimes act as if they don't exist; you'll never come to any grief by disregarding them—up to a point, only it's impossible to fix that point. All doctors learn this eventually. They learn there is nothing absolutely safe in the world of medical practice, nothing that is not subject to the law of "up to a point." Much of medicine is balanced on that cornerstone. Many doctors follow rules, guidelines, and algorithms, and by doing so they hope to get through an entire career unscathed. They want to hear, "It is forbidden to do this," or "It is the duty of the doctor to do that"—the kind of straightforward counsel that comes with rules and guidelines. They prefer not only to be given direction but also to be made aware of the penalties for not following that direction, and to have the magnitude of those penalties defined beforehand. Then they discover that rules and guidelines come with exceptions and gray areas that *they* are responsible for navigating through. This scares them.

Practicing medicine is about *living in a state of fear*, in the knowledge that rules must be followed but only "up to a point," and what that point is a doctor never knows for sure. Doctors hope in their imaginations that someone will tell them what that point is, that a colleague will say, "Don't worry, this is one of those exceptions to the rule. Ignore the rule," or "If you follow the rule, you may suffer a penalty, but at most that penalty will be a small misfortune," or "On this one you'd better follow the rule." But doctors hope in vain. They are sentenced to fear, often, and at a moment's notice, for rules exist everywhere in medicine, to guide them, but also to worry them, to paralyze them, and possibly to ruin them. Some doctors recognize it is useless to try to define what "up to a point" means, and that there's nothing a doctor can do about it other than wallow in a bog of insecurity. They just ignore the contradiction and let the chips fall where they may. Some reputable doctors think this way, although so do many physician-cowboys. Other doctors just live in fear.

I thought about what drug I might use for spinal anesthesia. The case was scheduled for two hours, so I needed something that lasted longer than lidocaine. Bupivicaine seemed like the best choice. Because Ms. O would be lying on her side with her broken hip up during the operation, it made sense to use a preparation called "normobaric bupivicaine." When injected, the drug numbs a patient on both sides, no matter what position the patient is in, unlike "hyperbaric bupivicaine," which settles down by gravity and numbs the down side preferentially. Normobaric spinal bupivicaine exists in the form of straightforward epidural bupivicaine. Curiously, the label on the bottle reads (to this day), "Not to be used for spinal blocks"; yet I thought for sure I had seen other anesthesiologists use it for spinal anesthesia. I asked another anesthesiologist about it.

"I'm pretty sure you can use it for a spinal. The label is leftover from the old days, when they thought these solutions were neurotoxic. They know that's not the case now," he said.[1]

"Then why didn't they change the label?" I asked. I kept staring at the label and the rule printed on it: "Not to be used for spinal blocks." I felt uneasy. Like the platelet rule, it hypnotized me, although it was supposedly no longer a rule.

"I guess the FDA forgot to. Listen, the rule must have been crazy, even in the old days, because you always risk accidentally injecting some anesthetic into the spinal canal when placing an epidural. So even when they thought the drug was neurotoxic, they still allowed it," he replied.

"This is idiotic," I complained.

"You're right. It is idiotic. But there's nothing you can do about it. You see, the system is idiotic," he said.

"Wait, you know the system is idiotic. So then why don't doctors change the system?" I asked.

"They can't," he said. "But that's okay, because the system is idiotic and I live under the system, but it doesn't oblige me to be an idiot. And other doctors aren't idiots, either. Everyone understands everything, but there's nothing they can do."

Eager to elude the more obvious danger, and now flummoxed by a label, I surrendered to the power of the platelet rule and opted for general anesthesia.

I gave Ms. O two puffs of her asthma inhaler and brought her into the operating room, While the patient breathed oxygen on her own, the nurse announced a time-out. Everyone in the room stopped what they were doing and paid attention, as required during a time-out. Afterward I began the anesthetic induction.

Because Ms. O had eaten only a few hours before, I could not slowly breathe for her during the induction to get her deep on gas and in that way lessen the chance of bronchospasm associated with intubation. Mask ventilation risks churning up a patient's stomach contents and causing aspiration. Instead, I rapidly injected the anesthetic drugs into her intravenous and intubated her. Then I connected the breathing tube to the anesthesia circuit and squeezed the bag.

Tremendous resistance kept me from pushing air into her lungs. I listened to high-pitched squeaks in Ms. O's chest with my stethoscope as I compressed the bag with all my strength. She was in bronchospasm. Her oxygen saturation dropped. The pressure needed to push air into her lungs was high enough to risk pneumothorax. I quickly turned on the anesthetic agent to dilate her bronchi, but it was hard to get air into her lungs, let alone anesthetic agent. Meanwhile, the nurse announced a second time-out.

When time-outs were first introduced, some doctors and nurses grumbled that they delayed the start of a case. Nevertheless, these providers adapted, especially when they realized the time-out's safety benefits. Some hospitals, however, doubled down on the time-out, or even tripled down on it. They demanded staff perform two time-outs or even three time-outs before starting a case, thinking that if one time-out decreased the rate of medical error, more time-outs would do so even more. In other words, although doctors invented the idea of the time-out, administrators took control of the idea and ran with it. Doubling and tripling the number of time-outs is not illogical, at least theoretically. But it does push against the law of diminishing returns.

The nurse announcing the second time-out demanded my attention. During a time-out all staff must stop what they are doing and listen. But I was busy managing Ms. O's bronchospasm. The nurse asked me to stop and pay attention. I told her I was busy. The nurse hesitated over what to do next. Should she ask me again to stop? Should she skip the second time-out? Should she continue with the time-out while making an exception for me? She fidgeted for a few seconds, during which time I recognized the anxiety in her eyes. It was the same anxiety that I had about the platelet rule. A rule in medicine demands certain conduct; if you violate that rule, you risk getting into trouble. In my case, I feared a lawsuit; in her case, she feared being fired. The time-out rule was the rule at most hospitals, rigidly enforced, "up to a point," but what that point was she didn't know.

I wanted to help her. I wanted to tell her that doctors had invented the time-out rule, and that because I was a doctor I knew the exact point when the rule could be overlooked. But we doctors had lost control of the time-out rule, just as we had lost control of the platelet rule. Hospital administrators now owned the rule, and there was nothing I could do. Fortunately, the nurse made the sensible decision and conducted the time-out without me.

I broke Ms. O's bronchospasm with inhalers and anesthetic gas. With difficulty we moved Ms. O onto her side, almost three-quarters prone. The nurse prepped the patient's hip and the surgeon started to cut.

An hour into the surgery I noticed the pressure needed to push air into Ms. O's lungs rising again. I listened to her chest but heard no wheezing. The pressure continued to rise. I turned off the ventilator and manually squeezed air into her lungs with great difficulty. Thinking there might be an obstruction in the breathing tube itself, I passed a suction catheter through it. The catheter barely passed. Out through the catheter flowed thick yellow, gelatinous mucus. The breathing tube's presence had likely precipitated these thick secretions.

I needed an extra pair of hands to help me suction out the breathing tube. I looked over to the circulating nurse, but she was sitting on a stool, her back toward me, entering data on the computer. She had been entering data since the start of the case. It wasn't her fault. New rules nationwide demanded that operating room nurses enter enormous amounts of data, to be collated later by administrators and policymakers to make more rules. The goal was medical safety. And yet time-consuming data entry often robs the operating room of a nurse's observant mind and skilled hands at a crucial moment. Rather than decrease the risk of catastrophe, it sometimes raises it.

A few minutes later the breathing tube obstructed almost completely.

"We have to turn the patient back on her back—now! I need to re-intubate her," I said excitedly.

"But I'm in the middle of the operation," pleaded the surgeon.

"I don't care. We have an airway emergency. Just cover the operative site with a sterile drape," I insisted.

The surgeon reluctantly draped the site. The nurse turned her head away from the computer screen. She looked as though she had only just been awakened from sleep and opened her eyes wide, trying to grasp the situation. Quickly she refocused. Since the operating table was too narrow for us to maneuver Ms. O back onto her back, the nurse ran out the door to get the stretcher we had brought her in on. The plan was to jam the stretcher next to the operating table to give us a larger platform on which to turn the patient over.

But the stretcher was gone! I was furious. A rescue stretcher was supposed to sit outside the door for just this problem. The nurse panted out what had happened: a new rule in the fire code had demanded that all halls in hospitals be cleared of stretchers. I told the nurse to go find another stretcher. Ms. O's oxygen saturation dropped lower. Her color grew dusky. I had no choice but to remove her breathing tube with her lying on her side and try to breathe for her with her face half-buried in a pillow.

It was an almost impossible task. The pillow pressed up against the side of her face and kept me from securing a tight mask fit. Secretions poured out of her mouth, wetting both the mask and my gloves, and causing the mask to slip from my grip. Also, her tongue obstructed her airway. With my left hand holding the mask, I stretched out with my right hand toward the instrument table to grab an oral airway. It was there—but wrapped in plastic. A new rule required all airways to be wrapped in plastic bags. The rule seemed silly to me, as the airways were run through a sterilizer and therefore were more sterile than any patient's mouth. But I had already been reprimanded once for violating the rule. A rule is a rule, "up to a point," but what that point was I never knew, so I just followed the rule.

I dropped the mask and grabbed the oral airway. Then I used my wet, gloved hands to tear open the plastic. This took time, during which Ms. O's oxygen saturation dropped lower.

I put the oral airway inside Ms. O's mouth and breathed for her just as the nurse rushed in with the new stretcher. We tilted Ms. O's body toward the stretcher, making it easier for me to mask ventilate her. Her oxygen level returned to normal. Still, I needed to re-intubate her to keep her from aspirating her stomach contents. To do so I needed more muscle relaxant, which sat inside the new anesthesia carts that had mandatory locks. Before, such drugs had been available in open drawers. Administrators around the country had decided this was wrong because it meant drugs could be stolen or go unaccounted for. Carts with locks took over. I always distrusted the locks for fear they would jam during the worst possible moment, as during an emergency, and so I got in the habit of keeping emergency drugs in my scrub shirt pocket. In particular, I would keep an ampule of Versed on me while working in obstetrics so that I could treat a patient suffering from an eclamptic seizure. The four minutes needed to chase down Versed in a locked cart could be catastrophic in such an emergency. But the new rule didn't allow for exceptions, and rather than test the rules by hiding one or two drugs in my pocket, I went bare. I had no muscle relaxant on me when the lock jammed in Ms. O's case.

A bureaucrat had written the rule on locked carts. And the rule did have the flavor of truth. Some drugs do go unaccounted for. The bureaucrat had written the rule in good faith. But there is often a divergence between words and things; a rule written down on paper fails to represent with sufficient exactitude the complexity of situations that might arise and invalidate that rule.

Why would an anesthesiologist follow this insane rule and not keep emergency drugs in his or her pocket? Because a normal person understands it is dangerous and pointless to oppose universal insanity, and rational to participate in it. In theory I was a doctor, but in reality I was an employee who lived in constant awareness that at any time I could be discovered, discussed, and punished. Doctors sometimes do ignore insane rules. They observe the rules only outwardly, while in fact living a semi-underground life. For example, anesthesiologists will write drug names on syringes but sometimes skip writing the time and date on them, thinking it silly to add such data when they'll be using the syringes a few minutes later. They will also remove their mandatory goggles before trying to intubate a patient with a difficult airway, to gain a better view. Although they do not challenge the authorities openly, they refuse to observe all accepted rituals, believing that some rules need only be followed "up to a point," with their judgment telling them what that point is.

However, most rules they do follow. In the past, doctors would not have been punished for exercising their judgment. Indeed, there was no one to punish them, since most doctors were self-employed independent professionals. Nowadays, most doctors are employed, and so they are punished. For an employed doctor to openly flout the rules is arguably insane.

I banged hard against the cart with my gloved hands that were wet with Ms. O's secretions. A new rule obligated me to change my gloves before touching the cart to prevent the spread of germs. But I didn't have time to change gloves! Worse, my hands were sweaty, and every experienced health care worker knows that putting gloves on wet, sweaty hands is a difficult and time-consuming process. The glove rule had no known exceptions. Nevertheless, I said to hell with rules.

I retrieved the drug from the cart. After giving Ms. O a few puffs of oxygen, I dropped the facemask and used both hands to draw up the muscle relaxant in a syringe. Then I dropped the syringe to give Ms. O another puff. Then I exchanged the mask for the syringe and removed the needle. I looked for a port in the intravenous line to inject the drug. A small secondary intravenous line occupied the port. I tried twisting it off, but the nurse had wedged it in too securely. I put the needle back on the syringe and looked for a port that would accept needles. There was none. A new rule had banned such ports, thinking such ports encouraged the use of needles, which were said to be unsafe. A nurse rushed over with a hemostat to help me twist off the line stuck in the lone port. In the meantime I gave Ms. O a few extra puffs. Unfortunately, as the nurse twisted, the line broke off just above the point of insertion, rendering the port blocked and useless. I gave Ms. O another puff. The nurse and I rushed to replace the intravenous line with a new one. I gave Ms. O two more puffs. When the new line was in place I injected the muscle relaxant and re-intubated Ms. O.

I should have done a spinal.

The rest of the case proceeded uneventfully, until, as we wheeled Ms. O to the recovery room, I realized that I had failed to relock the anesthesia cart. A rule demanded that I do so, and if an inspector had caught me abandoning an unlocked cart, I risked my job. I knew the inspectors from a hospital accreditation agency were due for a visit. Were they here now? I wondered. I stopped in the middle of the hallway; the nurse at the foot of the stretcher stared at me quizzically while I pondered what to do. If I abandoned Ms. O for the one minute needed to go back and lock the cart, I risked violating a rule. If I kept going toward the recovery room and left the cart unlocked, I risked violating another rule. In the end, I decided to drop Ms. O off in the recovery room first, and then circle back to lock the cart. My hand-off to the recovery room nurses was much faster than usual, though, as I kept worrying about whether the inspectors were around.

Rules in medicine are the creations of the doctors' inner selves. Doctors devise them in labs and research centers. They do so to improve medical safety. But doctors have lost control of their creations. Their creations have risen up against them. Malpractice lawyers own them. Hospital administrators own them. Accreditation agencies own them. Government agencies own them. As a result, doctors today fear their own creations. When they see a book of rules and guidelines, a mysterious voice whispers in their ears, "That's where 'up-to-a-point' lives." The rules must be followed, except when they should not be followed; only that critical inflection point is never revealed to them.

More rules and guidelines are written all the time. Almost every activity in medical practice has been carefully tabulated. Nothing has been overlooked; nothing has escaped the eye of researchers. There are detailed instructions for everything. But the new owners of these instructions have less feel for them than the doctors who created them do. They wrongly see them as information, something with a clear right and wrong, like an irrefutable math demonstration, something that comes with a sure path toward success. They do not see that rules and guidelines are only an approximation of truth, and that at every step they need a doctor's considered judgment to make them more exact.

Doctors, for their part, follow the rules, especially employed doctors who fear being sued *and* fired. The rules guide their decisions. Yet the rules also stand in the way of their decisions. Doctors love their rules, but at the same time they feel as if something terrible has been imposed on them. It has.

The inspectors from the hospital accreditation agency arrived a week later. Because hospitals would go out of business without recertification, doctors and hospital administrators fear them. Doctors are warned not to argue with them, to be polite and friendly, and to accept all their recommendations.

The inspectors entered my operating room while I set up for my case. Although neither inspector was a doctor, both looked confident in the operating room. They were the kind of people who are appointed to inspect and without a twinge of doubt will inspect firmly and decisively whatever it is they have been appointed to inspect, whether it be an operating room, an industry, or a school.

They studied my workspace. A laryngoscope blade lying half outside its package caught the main inspector's eye.

"What's this?" he asked in an icy tone.

"I always keep a blade half open, so as to be available in case of an airway emergency," I replied, my left eye twitching from nervousness.

"You don't keep it lying around all day? Correct?" the inspector asked sternly.

"Oh, no, of course not," I replied, although I knew anesthesiologists had been doing so for fifty years without problems.

Next, an open bottle of drug caught the main inspector's attention. I had drawn the drug up for my next patient but had yet to throw the bottle away, thinking I might need more.

"I assume you will use this bottle for your next patient only?" asked the inspector.

Although doctors have been using multi-dose vials on different patients for years, a new rule banned the practice to prevent infection. The rule was reasonable and I meticulously followed it, except once. I had needed the drug Pitocin to control hemorrhaging in an obstetrical patient whose uterus failed to contract after delivery. My anesthesia cart jammed and kept me from getting a new bottle. The only Pitocin available was in the bottle that I had used on the previous patient (but which was still sterile). I wanted to use it, but the rule momentarily hypnotized me. I hesitated for several seconds while my patient almost bled to death; then I said to hell with the rule and gave her the Pitocin. The drug saved her life. Still, I felt uneasy for having violated the rule.

"That's correct," I replied nervously. "One bottle, one patient."

The main inspector saw an unlabeled syringe containing the milky white drug Diprivan. I had drawn the drug up a few minutes before to use on my next patient.

"Why isn't this syringe labeled?" he growled.

"I just drew it up, so I know what it is. Besides, it's the only milky white drug we use, you know, so there's no chance of me confusing it with another drug, " I replied with confidence.

I could tell by the inspector's face that he didn't find my argument convincing.

"The drug could be Milk of Magnesia. That's milky white," said the main inspector with a straight face.

"Oh, come on," I giggled. "We don't use Milk of Magnesia in the operating room."

I looked for an ironic smile on the man's face, to see whether he was just pulling my leg. There was none. Instead, he glared at me, as if to say, "I represent a certain organization well known to you and I don't recommend you insult it. That would only make your position, bad as it is, worse."

"The rule is to label all drugs," he replied restrainedly, as if somehow offended. "Is that clear?"

He really was a natural-born predator. A passion lived within him, and he seemed to harbor the urge to hound and henpeck anyone weaker than he was. He would be happy to get me fired. The other inspector regarded me with more sympathy. Still, she expected a kind of respect to which she felt she was entitled as the representative of her agency. All good things came from her agency, meaning rules and guidelines that saved people's lives, and therefore good things should be given to her agency—in other words, respect. Although she didn't want to hurt me, her eyes suggested that if I continued to resist, I might become the unfortunate victim of cruel administrative necessity.

I repented and put a label on the syringe.

Some medical writers believe doctors today are so bombarded by information that they risk overlooking things, resulting in catastrophes.[2] These writers preach rules and protocols that help remind doctors to check this and remember that. But in my experience, although there is real value in rules and protocols, medical catastrophes stem less from doctors being flooded with information than from doctors being flooded with rules and protocols. Not necessarily with a checklist or a time-out, not necessarily with the rule to label all syringes, but with the hundreds of rules and protocols that collectively guide doctors in everyday medical practice and that should be followed, but only "up to a point." It is not the rules and protocols per se that cause catastrophe so much as doctors having lost control of those rules and protocols to higher-ups—to administrators, to inspectors, to bureaucrats, and to civil servants—who prevent doctors from judiciously applying them. Those higher-ups lurk in hospital corridors, fire orders at subordinates at point-blank range, sort out patient lives with the latest rules and protocols, and then stroll away. Deprived of an opportunity to use their own judgment about when to enforce the rules, doctors become little more than clerks. When the inner voice of judgment does whisper inside of them, they find it hard to think, because they are afraid; their minds go around and around in a vicious circle; they see a rule on one side and a threat on the other; they make decisions, sometimes senseless ones, in a state of vertigo. Employed doctors feel the most pressure.

In one case on the West Coast that I am familiar with, an obstetrician admitted a patient with gestational diabetes to an intensive care unit. Employed by the hospital, the intensivist insisted on giving the patient a flu shot, since a rule mandated that all patients with diabetes get flu shots. "But it's not diabetes, it's gestational diabetes," the obstetrician pleaded. "It's different." The obstetrician wanted to keep her patient from being needlessly exposed to the potentially dangerous complications of flu shots. But the intensivist feared being fired if he ignored the rule.

In a second case, an employed obstetrician rejected an anesthesiologist's suggestion that a patient with mild placenta previa be crossmatched for blood instead of just screened for blood.[3] Only with a crossmatch is blood immediately available for transfusion in case of severe hemorrhage. The obstetrician worried that the more expensive crossmatch would raise her financial profile and make her a statistical outlier among other employed obstetricians. The hospital had its protocol for managing such cases; a bureaucrat had estimated in advance the reasonable cost. If the obstetrician went outside that protocol and incurred a higher cost per case, she risked her job.

In a third case, an employed anesthesiologist hesitated to give her diabetic patient insulin before surgery, worrying that her patient, who was sensitive to the drug, might suffer a dangerous and undetectable drop in blood sugar during the operation. The hospital diabetes protocol, working from a nationwide protocol, had decreed insulin to be given when the blood sugar reached a certain number. The anesthesiologist hesitated. She didn't want to ignore the rule, but she feared losing her job.

Why bureaucracies put doctors in such an uncomfortable position mystifies physicians. Some doctors see a pernicious ploy to award them responsibility without authority. The bureaucracy lays down a rule. If doctors follow the rule and get a bad outcome, they get into trouble because the rule should have been followed "up to a point," and they should have known that point. If doctors ignore the rule and get a bad outcome, they get into trouble for not having followed the rule.

A more likely explanation lies in the nature of bureaucracy itself. An analogy is helpful. Imagine sitting in a theater and watching the actions of others. We are interested in the movie; what unfolds before us is familiar; the feelings that the actors express are familiar; and after the movie we talk about what the characters might have done differently. Yet, despite all that takes place on screen, no decision is required of us. The drama takes place in an imaginary world, and nothing we say or do has any real effect on that world. Real patient care is a kind of imaginary world for bureaucrats. Bureaucrats think and talk about that world. They feel for people in that world. That world is familiar to them. They may even have once worked in that world. Yet patient care is still a distant world that fails to touch them directly. The major difference between a bureaucrat's relationship to his imaginary world and a moviegoer's relationship to his imaginary world is that, for the bureaucrat, decisions *do* affect the imaginary world. Sometimes bureaucrats forget this fact. When writing rules for patient care, they use words, flimsy symbols, and sometimes forget the terrible consequences that may follow. Their words or phrases fail to represent with sufficient exactitude what happens in the patient care world and the consequences of following them. The result can be catastrophe.

Ironically, the medical profession is responsible for this bad situation. Under the old model of doctoring that guided my father, physicians did not have the same obsession with rules, protocols, and algorithms. True, my father worked with rules and protocols, and he often followed them. But for him the underlying difference between doctors was less one of who knew the rules and more a matter of personal taste. My father believed that in delicate and difficult matters of patient care, individual variations of temperament and personality among doctors were really the dominant elements in any judgment. This was the "gentlemanly," almost aristocratic side to medical practice.

In contrast, many doctors today fear individual variation among themselves as much as they fear not having a ready answer for patients. The idea that they should manage illness not through universal rules and protocols but through personal experience and a half-conscious sense of the vital elements in a situation unnerves some doctors. These doctors embrace habit. They want to fall into routine. They want to reduce the effect of human variation among doctors. They want science to smooth out the fluctuations between them. They want "best practice" guidelines. They want a rule to tell them what to do.

Their hopes and fears have led to an explosion in the number of rules and protocols in medicine. Those rules and protocols are now dangerously under the control of higher-ups.

9

THE PROBLEM OF GOING PART-TIME
AND WHEN TO RETIRE

December. Late at night. Cold and tired. My first year in practice. On the other side of the ether screen the surgeon sliced off the patient's appendix. I tickled the roof of my mouth with my tongue to stay awake, a trick I had learned as an intern. To pass the time, I studied my patient's face.

An anesthetic-induced sleep does not convey an image of peace. On the contrary, it conveys an image of fear. The cheeks are pale. The veins at the temples stick out repugnantly. The bloodshot eyes fasten their gaze on one spot, unblinkingly, as if aware of some invisible approaching horror. The hair is busy, hectic, and dank with sweat. Even the nicest nose is snotty, as if the owner were too harried to wipe it. When watching someone in real sleep, one has a sense of life reviving, that sleep is a good thing, that a tired spirit is putting forth fresh shoots. When watching someone in an anesthetized sleep, one has a sense of life in despair. Horrible thoughts seem to reveal themselves on the patient's face. The damp forehead; the cold, bloodless lips; the tearing eyes; the mouth in the shape of a groan—all suggest that the world is getting worse and worse to live in.

When the case finished I went back to my call room to lie down. Although the day-shift physician had been there only a few hours, the room looked and smelled as though someone had been living there, sleeping and eating his meals there, for over a year. An unmade bed. A Styrofoam cup filled with old coffee. From the trashcan came the noxious smell of rotting tuna salad. Within a few seconds my nose adjusted to the bad odor; yet I knew I wouldn't sleep well in this stale, stuffy room. I sat down on the unmade bed, took off my cap, then my shoes, giving my feet a chance to feel their freedom. I unwrapped my stethoscope from around my neck and put it on the table. I wondered if I should take off my scrubs before commencing my hours-long stare into the darkness. It seemed senseless to get undressed for that pleasure—not really to sleep, just to lie down on a dirty bed and stare.

Lying alone in a call room is a special time for doctors. It is the moment when the mind is irresistibly attuned to dreams, the heart to all those sensations that in the light of everyday life seem silly, absurd, even juvenile. It is also the moment when the doctor ceases to be active, when boredom lies in wait for him, when he is prey to imaginary worries, endless self-examination, regret for the past, and fears for the unknown future.

The memory of my patient's despairing face set the tone for the evening. Simply put, I was unhappy with being a doctor. I wasn't sure why. It certainly wasn't the money. Both my father and my grandfather had loved being doctors, and my father, at least, had earned a good living, but compared to what I was earning (even in my first year of practice) they were practically paupers.

Some of my disappointment stemmed from the monotony of anesthesia practice. Ninety percent of the time I would give a patient all the big syringe (the Pentothal), then all the little syringe (the muscle relaxant), insert a breathing tube, and turn the knob on the gas canister. In my early years of training I had a feeling of excited expectation in learning how to do this. By my last year of residency this cooled considerably. During the first six months of private practice it came with an ironic smile. In the second six months it was transformed into indifference.

Overspecialization has caused many doctors today to share in this feeling of monotony. Wherever they are, the weather outside will have changed, their watches will have moved ahead, but their day is exactly the same as the one they had three weeks before. They did all this yesterday and the day before, and they know they will do the very same thing tomorrow and after. They grow depressed in spirit; they are overcome at the assembly line with a daily state of madness that lasts for ten hours, after which, upon returning home, they rest, eat well, get well, and recuperate, in order on the next day again to grow mad for a while.

Yet both my father and my grandfather often did the same thing every day, and they enjoyed being doctors. Indeed, most work is monotonous. Perhaps my career expectations had been too high, based on fabrications of television shows. Real medical practice, like real life, was something different—boring and simpler—and I would simply have to submit to it.

I lay on my bed and listened. The hospital murmured vaguely. I heard the sound of an elevator opening, the sniff of someone next door, and the rumble of a toilet flushing down the hall. Then came a severe silence, waiting to be pierced by a beeper's staccato ring, that harbinger of disaster, alerting a doctor to some patient in distress. At home, dogs bark, kids scream, jackhammers pound away in the street, and yet sleep is easy; while at the hospital, silence is almost total, one can practically hear two clouds colliding in the sky, and yet sleep is hard—all because of that little beeper sitting two feet from one's head, waiting to go off like a time bomb and putting a tremendous strain on the nerves. Nothing is more irritating than being awakened by that beeper. It is more painful than doing the entire case for which one is awakened.

If the position of "doctor" had been more respected, then my discomfort might have been more endurable. But it had ceased to be. It had been respected during my father and grandfather's time. It is why the two men never said they were "retired" whenever people asked them during their final years what they did. Like the general who calls himself a general long after having left the army, my father and grandfather said they were doctors long after they had stopped practicing. They clung to the title. Being a doctor was a high-status position in those days, and they were proud of it, while society's respect got them through the long hours. In a game called Life that I played as a child, the position of doctor was the highest a player could attain, and came with the highest salary, followed (in order) by lawyer, journalist, and teacher. Even in the early 1980s, when I went to medical school, the brightest young people often aspired to the professions. But later, an entirely new upper stratum came into being, composed of people in finance, computers, the Internet, media, entertainment, and high technology. Indeed, in today's version of Life, the position of doctor has no high rank, the job of computer consultant or entertainer comes with more perks, and salaries are awarded at random. A doctor my age, shell-shocked by the change, once confided in me, "A doctor is nothing."

A noise outside the room distracted me. I looked at the light coming from a crack at the bottom of the door to check for any divots of shade caused by feet, but I saw none. I settled back down once I realized that it was just the cleaning lady, the wheels on her laundry cart squeaking as they rolled down the corridor, with the woman herself muttering in bad-tempered irritation about some injustice that had been done to her.

I felt embarrassed. Obviously, the cleaning lady's life was harder than my own. So what if doctoring is just any old job? It brings no glory, but it also brings no great misery. "Where's my gratitude?" I had asked. Well, there was none. I should be satisfied and at peace, as if I had achieved everything I had dreamed of. I was living a normal life.

I wanted my beeper to go off at that moment. Time to get up, work, live. But it didn't. Inevitably my mind drifted toward other complaints. Professional medicine calls the doctor a master technician. But I wanted to talk to someone about culture, about higher things, about the eternal. Technicians don't talk about such things. Professional medicine calls the doctor a scientist. *That's a stretch*, I thought. As a student I had watched orthopedic surgery residents perform an experiment that involved break-ing bunny rabbits' legs and putting them in slings. When I raised an eyebrow, the residents said defensively, "Hey, we're scientists. We're MDs." I replied sarcastically, "So what do the plastic surgery residents do? Give the bunnies a 'boob' job?" Nuclear physicists they were not. Professional medicine calls the doctor a gentleman. Yet when business turned medical practice into an assembly line, many doctors no longer even had time to eat lunch. Some anesthesiologists smuggled food into their operating rooms as a wretched substitute—not celery or apples, since the crunching sound might alert the authorities, but candy bars and bananas. The doctor is a gentleman? Even the lowliest animal in a cage gets lunch.

Professional medicine calls the doctor a professional. But a profes-sional is in control of his personality. An employed doctor has no such control. The company owns his smiles, his demeanor, and his language, for these have commercial significance; they affect doctor-patient rela-tions. Alone in the call room at night is the only time when a doctor is not pretending for anyone.

Professional medicine calls the doctor a benefactor, someone who sacrifices himself for the good of others. But I didn't go into medicine to sacrifice myself. I did think about my happiness: *Where's my happiness?*

I asked myself. Something was working against my happiness, and it made me angry. Nature was rising up within me, seeking to reassert some universal rule that had been violated. I had read philosophers who said that all happiness is built on empty space, a feeling that had no basis. I disagreed. *Everyone wants to be happy. Can't they understand? No one can rid himself of the want*, I thought.

Frightened by my own discontent, I switched on the light and picked up a journal. Then I felt sleepy. I knew that if I put down the journal and turned off the light, the feeling would be gone. I switched on the television. I half-watched a documentary, then decided you either watch a documentary properly or not all, and turned it off. I lay there and dreamed of dancing and singing. *Don't be impatient, happiness will come*, I said to myself. *You won't be in this call room forever. When the time comes, happiness will come. Happiness is everywhere, in everything.*

Then I stood up and looked in the mirror. At first glance I looked like an anesthetized patient, pale and despairing. Then I studied my face more carefully. I had the pallor of the person whose working day is not regulated and too often goes beyond midnight, of the person who has no time for indulgence in sports, of the person who eats any old way. I was unshaved; my hair was uncombed. In a word, here was a man who worked too hard, who no longer cared for anything at all, and who merely continued to drag out his existence. A tired man—tired of his work, himself, his thoughts, his doubts. And yet I was only thirty-one years old.

My youth had been lost somewhere in the smoke of time, never to return, never to come to life again in the green grass and sunshine. Even now, precious minutes were flying. Something turned over inside me, the last barrier, the last thread attaching me to a conventional medical career. I decided that very soon I would go part-time.

I met Dr. B while in training. In his early forties, he had gone part-time at a young age to enjoy life and see the world. A part-time doctor was a rarity in those days. It was also frowned upon. Many doctors called being part-time childish. Some said it showed a lack of dedication to the profession. A few said it was dangerous. But Dr. B didn't care. When he saw some female doctors going part-time to raise their children, he decided to go part-time for no other purpose than to escape medicine's hellish work hours and live a balanced life.

We were paged to the emergency room, where an elderly man was diagnosed with a leaking abdominal aortic aneurysm. It was the ultimate vascular emergency. The great vessel leaving the man's heart had a defect in its wall as it descended through the abdominal cavity. The wall now had a hole in it. Blood was leaking out. If the aneurysm ruptured, the man would hemorrhage to death in two minutes.

Dr. B looked nervous. His eyes darted like a lemur's. He had just come off a two-month stint hiking in Europe, and he hadn't done a surgical case in all that time. When the patient arrived on the operating table he raced to apply the blood pressure cuff and EKG pads. He was keyed up, but also distracted and rough. He seemed to want to be done with this operation, to be sitting upstairs in the cafeteria and laughing about the final resolution to this nightmare, which was still open-ended and in the future. It was almost as if he resented the patient for having ruined his afternoon.

Dr. B injected two drugs into the man's intravenous. Twenty seconds passed between the moment of injection and the man's loss of consciousness, during which time the whole room fell quiet and still. Dr. B placed the breathing tube, then listened to the characteristic sound in the man's chest as he squeezed air into it.

Thirty seconds later an alarm went off on the machine. No blood pressure was obtainable. Dr. B cycled the machine again, his eyes growing wider with concern. Again the alarm sounded.

"Everything all right?" asked the surgeon.

"Yeah, just wait a minute," Dr. B replied impatiently. "I think something's wrong with the machine."

"Should I do anything?" asked the surgeon.

"No, just wait a minute, will you?" Dr. B barked nervously. A shrewd nurse quietly paged another anesthesiologist to come help.

The patient's pallor had turned a ghostly white; his lips were barely distinguishable from the rest of his skin. A third attempt at getting a blood pressure proved futile. Now terrified, his pupils enormous, Dr. B reached for a drug to artificially raise the man's pressure. He was about to inject it when another anesthesiologist, Dr. V, burst into the room. When she saw everyone standing around flummoxed, and then saw the patient's deathly pallid face, she instinctively knew what had happened.

"Cut him!" she shouted.

"What?" asked the surgeon.

"Cut him!"

Dr. V saw the patient's bare, unprepped abdomen.

"Dr. B!"

Dr. B stood still, frozen in place by fear, his eyes fixed attentively on Dr. V, the gaze of a frightened animal. He dared not even to blink.

"Dr. B! Get the iodine solution!" Dr. V raced past him, grabbed the bottle of orange-brown iodine, and squirted it furiously over the man's abdomen. Then she lunged past Dr. B to grab two large-bore intravenous catheters from the anesthesia cart. Dr. B stood aside, paralyzed, unsure what to do, although eager to defend his actions to Dr. V.

"I didn't give that much Pentothal. If his blood pressure dropped from the Pentothal, it's not my fault," Dr. B whispered intensely. He stared at Dr. V with entreaty and hatred in his eyes.

"It wasn't the Pentothal, you numbskull. He's hemorrhaging," whispered Dr. V with equal intensity, making sure no one else could hear. "You think this guy drove two hours to the hospital, made it to the emergency room, made it to the elevator, made it to the operating room, and then, just by coincidence, lost his blood pressure the moment you started giving anesthesia? No, your muscle relaxant weakened the outside pressure containing the aneurysm, causing it to explode. The patient should have been prepped and draped, with blood units already in the room, before you even started." Then Dr. V shouted, "Someone, call for blood!"

"When you grab hold of his aorta, squeeze tight until we get some blood into him! Just clamp it and pray!" she yelled at the surgeon.

The race began. The surgeon began slicing the patient's abdomen with deep strokes, as if he were a butcher hacking meat, the patient's intestines pouring out of the wound, an intertwined mass still steaming with bodily heat but abnormally pale, limp, and bloodless, without the usual stirring and swelling motions of the bowel. A tongue of blood spurted out lizard-like from underneath the mass, and then blood began to ooze out all over. Large dark clots floating in a red current streamed over the sides of the wound onto the surgeon's feet and beyond onto the floor, leaving puddles for us to step in.

We placed two more intravenous catheters. Blood spread over my ungloved hands and fingernails, emitting a sickly sweet smell. As the surgeon hacked his way deeper into the man's belly, blood spattered everywhere, including onto the uncovered part of my face and neck.

The nurse called out, "The patient has no blood available. The specimen sent to the blood bank clotted, and so they couldn't do the cross-match."

"Are you serious?" the surgeon shouted, working furiously. "Come on! What the hell is going on here? No blood available for a major vascular case? Who forgot to check . . . ?"

"It doesn't matter," Dr. V interrupted, knowing it was probably Dr. B who had failed to follow up. Perhaps desiring to shield him from another blow, she told the surgeon, "We're going to need more blood than they would have typed for." Then she told the nurse, "Just send for as much Type O blood as they can give us."

Dr. B seemed to understand what Dr. V had done on his behalf. He slightly resented his weakness and Dr. V's reminder of it but said nothing, for he knew he had made another mistake.

Several minutes later the orderly lugged into the room a large box containing blood units. We transfused each unit as fast as we could.

Fifteen minutes later the patient's blood pressure returned to measurable levels, although his color still hovered menacingly between white and ash-gray. The surgeon held on to the patient's aorta as if it were a wriggling snake, waiting for more transfused blood to fill up the patient's vascular system. Still, the suction canisters roared, inhaling blood into their gaping maws. The blood pressure disappeared again—this time for good. The patient bled to death. We could not resuscitate him.

Part-time doctors are a new phenomenon in medicine. Before the 1990s, they were rare. By 2005, 7 percent of male doctors and 29 percent of female doctors were part-time. In 2011, 22 percent of male doctors and 44 percent of female doctors were part-time.[1] A doctor's desire to go part-time today is understandable. Medical training is longer than ever. Subspecialties such as cardiology and orthopedic surgery now need as many as eight years of postgraduate work, up from five years in 1970.[2] Many doctors today don't start living adult lives, with real salaries, until their late thirties. Naturally they feel impatience and regret, as I had in my call room. They want another life, and so they go part-time.

Other statistics hint at what is happening: In a 2014 survey, 60 percent of physicians older than forty-five had negative views toward being a doctor; yet almost 50 percent of physicians younger than forty-five shared the same negative views.[3] Young doctors today are surprisingly cynical and jaded about their profession. Their inward cursing and brooding inevitably leads many of them to go part-time; it's as if they want to remedy the mistake they made by going into medicine in the first place. Indeed, many older full-time doctors have left independent practice to become hospital employees, not because they like being employed, but because they are unable to find young doctors willing to join their practices and take night and weekend call, so determined are young doctors these days to live their lives.

Professional medicine remains quiet on this issue. It shouldn't. Part-time doctoring has the potential to increase the risk of catastrophes, as it affects a doctor's ability to retain vital instincts. Dr. B was a case in point.

Being a creature of habit is a bad thing in a physician. A doctor who follows rules and protocols unthinkingly can make bad decisions. Yet being a creature of habit is also a good thing in a physician. It helps turn conscious decision making into instinct. This makes a doctor safe.

A surgeon, for example, is often a creature of habit. He will often eat the same breakfast at the same time every morning and stand on the same side of the operating table every day because he prefers to work reflexively, almost without thinking, with no new feeling in his mind, his hands, his stomach, or his bladder to perturb him. It is why a surgeon can work after being awake for forty hours; too tired to think, he works by habit, which is how he works best. Even a surgeon's lashing out in anger is more of a habit than an action, as a rude surgeon is typically rude to everyone.

When the surgeon cuts, the choice of where and how to cut is sometimes not even conscious. The surgeon thinks with his fingers and his scalpel. This is vital to being a good surgeon. It is analogous to the boxer who thinks with his body. The boxer never has time to say to himself, "Since my opponent is doing this, I will do that." Instead, the boxer thinks with his arms and his gloves. If there is the smallest break in the motion, if it pauses only slightly while the boxer hesitates and reasons, the rhythm breaks down and the exercise becomes impossible. It is the same with a surgeon, who establishes a direct communication between his eyes fixed on the patient and his fingers holding the knife.

In medicine, the art of thinking is often the art of making thought instinctive. Instinctive thoughts have narrow limits, but they can be infallible—and lifesaving. It is through instinct, born of the thousands of cases he or she has observed, that a doctor acquires the flashing rapidity of decision that medical events sometimes require.

Part-time doctoring threatens such instincts. In Dr. B, principles that would have percolated quickly and naturally to the surface of consciousness in a full-time doctor were repressed. Had he been given time, he might have been able to conjure them up—for example, the need to prep and drape a patient with a leaking aneurysm before inducing anesthesia. But conjuring takes time, and he had none. Knowledge is a doctor's only if, at the moment of need, it offers itself to the mind without the need for long meditation, for which there is no time.

Anesthesiologists are also creatures of habit. When shown a new drug, an anesthesiologist sometimes thinks, "Let me not know about it; then I will be happy." This is a bad habit, as it prevents the anesthesiologist from learning new things. Yet vigilance to the point of suspicion is also a habit, and a good one. In the surgical theater every funny-looking face suggests to the anesthesiologist a difficult intubation, every operating room an ambush; every morbidly obese patient sends an unpleasant shudder down his spine. He looks at the patient and his first instinct is to think, "How can this patient ruin me?" An anesthesiologist learns during training that another person will leave you in the lurch, and not to trust anyone—that, for example, if a technician says the oxygen is turned on, look yourself to make sure it is turned on—and that such suspicion will never let you down; it will see you through everything and help you avoid getting into trouble. Such suspicion goes hand in hand with attention to detail, which helps prevent catastrophes. Dr. B had lost this habit, forgetting, for example, to check whether the blood bank had performed the necessary crossmatch.

Anesthesiologists often work on instinct more than on scientific knowledge. It is instinct that gets them through a tense situation when panic threatens to blot out their knowledge base. Anesthesiologists who work sporadically risk losing this instinct, much the way an animal, once domesticated, loses the instinct to survive in the wild. Not all part-time doctors, but some.

The result is a characteristic personality. Creeping into an operating room after having been away for many weeks, part-time anesthesiologists anxiously put their patients to sleep. When they succeed and everything goes smoothly, they are lulled into thinking that everything is easy, that they can put anyone to sleep, that their work is a no-brainer. Then, when catastrophe approaches, they swing to the opposite side and panic, thinking everything is impossible. Anesthesiologists with healthy instincts manage an impending catastrophe in stages, with each stage getting their attention—for example, in a trauma case, first take care of the airway, then take care of the breathing, then take care of the patient's circulation. They do not look further than each stage while concentrating on a particular stage; they are like the mountain climber who cuts steps in the ice and focuses on the level he is at, refusing to look up at the heights or down into the depths because the sight of either might distract him. Part-time anesthesiologists, however, are sometimes petrified by the enormity of the situation they face. They look at the whole situation, all at once, instead of trying to build themselves a path to safety, step by step; they look up and they look down, and grow terrified and paralyzed.

One solution to the problem of the part-time doctor is to prevent doctors from going part-time in the first place. But this is impossible. My father and grandfather saw being a doctor as something special. With the collapse of that vision, today's physicians look at being a doctor as a job. And once doctoring becomes a job, the lure of part-time is often too strong to resist.

Can anyone blame them? Many young doctors want to save themselves from a hellish life made up of long work hours and few happy moments. Some people try to make them feel guilty for wanting to go part-time, only why should they feel guilty? Yes, they're a little to blame, because of their strong sense of entitlement, but life itself is also to blame. They slave away at their jobs. Suddenly temptation comes their way. It sucks and sucks at them, drawing all the time, and they're supposed to turn it aside? That's the right turn in life? But how can that be? How can it be not to want to have a family and see that family grow up, or not to have time to read, or to think about something beyond medicine, or to bend down and smell the flowers? Many doctors in the past, including my father, took a half-day off every week. They often took their staff out for lunch. They didn't need to go part-time because medical practice in those days allowed them some wiggle room. Such civilities went by the wayside long ago. No, if a doctor's life is all work, monotonous work, little-respected work, and employed work, then life is just as much to blame for a doctor's desire to go part-time.

The only solution to the problem of the part-time doctor is to make sure that the doctor never goes part-time *in his or her mind*. Even when a part-time anesthesiologist is away from work, he must constantly run scenarios of difficult cases in his mind. Whether he's hiking in Europe or sailing on the bay, he must take time out from his activity to imagine what he might do in a particular case. He must give that case his full attention. He must be so in the moment of his daydream that his heart races with expectation when he imagines injecting the life-saving drug, while his fingers twitch as he imagines inserting an emergency intravenous. When out in the everyday world, he must look at passersby and study their facial anatomy and imagine how he might care for them if they arrived for surgery, and whether he might intubate them awake or asleep. He must carry his art with him wherever he goes during his time off. Like a shadowboxer who spars with an imaginary opponent, he must use his art constantly, daily, in his mind, so that when hospital life returns, his instincts and reflexes are ready to go.

I know this because I have been part-time now for more than twenty years.

An anesthesiologist lives a good life and earns quite a bit of money, but his life is overshadowed by fear. And for good reason. Odds are that sooner or later, no matter what, he'll kill a patient by accident. When he does, he is often traumatized, both by the death and by the inevitable lawsuit. This risk causes some anesthesiologists to dream of the day when they no longer have to go into a cold operating room and put patients to sleep, but instead can teach or do administrative work. Sometimes they dream of suffering the perfect injury—left arm weakness—that will put them on disability without sidelining them from tennis or golf.

An anesthesiologist's fear intensifies when he's handed the operating room schedule for the day. He quickly surveys it to see if he's posted to work in a room with sick patients, where the chance of killing someone is high. If so, his heart is gripped with fear of the impending clash; he has an inexplicable feeling of savage agitation, the kind that a soldier feels in the trenches, before the captain's whistle blows, sending him over the top and into battle. Sure enough, the surgical nurse will often shout over the lounge intercom, "We're going in!" to tell the anesthesiologist as he waits anxiously in his chair that his patient is being wheeled back to the operating room, and that the test of nerves is about to begin.

In the healthy anesthesiologist there is usually a period of inward transformation when he steels himself against what is to come and reminds himself that he can only do what he thinks is right. He goes over his plan again and feels himself equipped to carry it out. His fear starts to dissipate; he goes back to acting as if there are no dangers in medicine, or, if there are, he has never come to any grief by disregarding them. He walks toward the operating room with a clear mind.

An anesthesiologist who is about to retire—or who *needs* to retire— finds it hard to control such fear.

Dr. P was such a physician. In his early sixties, he had been a good anesthesiologist with a solid safety record, a pleasant colleague, and a happy man. But his partners began to notice a change in his personality. Something was bothering him. He grew less social. He would eat lunch in silence, as if afraid to look at others, afraid to reveal his inner thoughts. He became indifferent to everything, interested in nothing, and only wanted to be left in peace.

His behavior in the operating room also changed. He grew superstitious. After learning his room assignment he would hesitate to switch rooms with another doctor, as if thinking, "Perhaps the disastrous case to come is in my partner's room, and had I only stayed in the room that fate had decreed for me, I would have been fine. Then again, maybe the disastrous case to come is in my room, and if only I had done my partner a favor and switched, I would have avoided it." He would wrestle in his mind with what to do, go back and forth between the two different possibilities, and begin to hate the doctor who asked to make the switch, thinking him some kind of devil put on earth to trick him. Later, when setting up his workspace in the operating room, he would draw up every emergency drug in his cart as if it were insurance against needing them. It was as though he were playing some kind of cat-and-mouse game with destiny. When inducing anesthesia he would demand that everyone in the operating room be quiet. Staring angrily at the surgeon and nurse as they talked to each other about their weekend, he would mutter to himself, "Death is staring us in the eyes, and here you are chattering away about some trip to the beach."

The habits of a lifetime were disintegrating, and he was uncertain as he had never been before. Soon he began to have problems clinically. He was unable to intubate some easy patients. Maybe the light on the laryngoscope was dim, or maybe he was too fidgety, or maybe he took his eyes off the windpipe at the last minute, but in any event he couldn't get the tube in. Once, when another anesthesiologist came in to do it for him, he sent his stool flying, kicked it toward the cabinet, and flung the scope to the floor. Both the surgeon and the nurse in the room drew back in fright. Then Dr. P grew quiet, as though the violent behavior had released some pent-up truth from his heart.

One day, Dr. P was assigned to put a child to sleep for a tonsillectomy. Although I had just finished my shift, he asked me to stay a few extra minutes to talk about something. I shrugged my shoulders and agreed. Once we were in the operating room he picked up a few syringes and a laryngoscope and presented them to me, implying that I was expected to participate in this anesthetic and not simply listen to him talk. I grew suspicious and slightly resentful, but I grabbed the laryngoscope and began to breathe the child down with gas without bothering to ask Dr. P if that had been his plan. I had no doubts. Dr. P seemed relieved to have the instrument removed from his hand, and his face relaxed even more as I took over the case.

After the child was asleep, I looked over at Dr. P and asked, "Okay, what did you want to talk about?"

"Talk about?" asked Dr. P. He seemed confused.

"Yes, you said you wanted to talk to me about something."

Dr. P suddenly remembered his deception, and he replied, "Oh, well, it's late, why don't we just talk about it tomorrow?"

"Wait a minute. You said you wanted to talk."

Whatever relief Dr. P had felt from my presence passed into embarrassment, then into anger at having been found out. Suddenly he thundered:

"I said we'll talk about it tomorrow! I'm too tired to talk about it now!"

I flinched in surprise. "What are you boiling over like that for? You're the one who asked me. . . . Oh, forget it. Good-bye." I turned away in open dissatisfaction and walked out, angry at having been cheated out of a half-hour of time off.

I should have been more understanding. Dr. P needed to retire. If he continued working, he risked injuring a patient or even a catastrophe.

This phenomenon is not new in medicine, but changes in medicine have made it more of an issue. In my father and grandfather's time, a physician like Dr. P would have retired. The problem with older physicians in those days was different. Doctors then often loved being doctors. They loved all the trappings that went with being a doctor, from the free food at the hospital to the free pens given to them by drug company reps (indeed, after graduating medical school, a doctor need not buy a pen for the next fifty years). Doctoring defined their identities. Since doctors were typically independent professionals in those days, and since doctors often "covered" for one another, an impaired physician could cling to medical practice and continue working long after it was safe for him or her to do so, and risk causing a catastrophe. I know of two physicians in the 1980s, one with Parkinson's disease, another with early Alzheimer's, who severely injured patients because they refused to stop practicing medicine and no real mechanism existed to make them stop.

This is less of a problem now. Physicians increasingly are employed, and employers have no problem firing an impaired employee. In the past, hospitals were almost proud of their old doctors the way zookeepers are proud of their old lions. This is less the case now. For their part, physicians increasingly view their work as a job. They love doctoring less and are often happy to get out when they can.

Still, the indelicate subject of money will likely rear its ugly head in the future. With doctors employed and making less in salary, the question remains whether a doctor will have enough money to stop practicing when his or her career has begun its downward arc—in other words, when he or she has started to get scared of taking care of patients.

Some jobs recognize that workers cannot necessarily continue into their seventies without endangering the public. For example, firefighters are often pensioned off at fifty-five, since no one wants an elderly firefighter carrying them down a ladder from a burning window. Pilots face mandatory retirement at sixty-five. Already in their sixties, pilots must often be paired with younger copilots and undergo intensive medical screening. Still, these jobs force retirement because of presumed physical decline. Doctors, however, can be healthy physically while still showing important psychological signs of decline, especially fear, putting them at increased risk of causing a catastrophe. Nervous doctors who need to retire but who stick it out another five or ten years because they can't afford to do so present a new and ill-defined problem.

Dr. P retired shortly after our case together. I saw him several years later looking happy and like his old self again. When I asked him how his life had changed, he smiled and said, "Whenever I need a new pen now, I

have to buy one. Otherwise, I'm fine." He winked at me, and I understood.

10

I COME FULL CIRCLE

My patient was a forty-year-old obese man with a thick neck and an overbite, going for nasal surgery. I thought he might be a little hard to intubate, but I decided to put him to sleep in the routine way rather than place a breathing tube while he was still awake. I injected the Pentothal, then the short-acting muscle relaxant succinylcholine. Still, I was uneasy. I felt those brief seconds of inward tension that precede a tough intubation, when the pulse quickens in an anesthesiologist no matter how many patients he has put to sleep. The anesthesiologist feels an icy chill of loneliness, for once the drugs are given, only he stands between the patient and suffocation.

After the patient lost consciousness and stopped breathing, I looked into his mouth with my laryngoscope and searched for the windpipe. I saw nothing. I removed the scope and anxiously tossed it on my cart. Then I pressed the mask tightly against the patient's face with my left hand while my right hand squcezed the bag at my side. The patient's chest failed to rise. I pressed the mask harder. With the enormous tension in my fingers invisible, I looked like an anesthesiologist doing something completely natural, especially with my right hand collapsing the breathing bag every two seconds like clockwork. The nurse watching me probably thought my movements were directed by a cold, unemotional reason, so assured and confident they seemed. But my hand hurt and my palm sweated, while inside I experienced a premonition of disaster.

Grabbing the scope back, I tried to imagine the sudden crisis away. I peered into the patient's throat again, thinking, *I'm sure to reach the airway this time. Then everything will be fine, and I will go home like I do every day.* But I saw nothing. I removed the scope, inserted an oral airway, put the mask back on the patient's face, and squeezed the bag again with my right hand, furiously, as though I were squeezing a bellows to start a fire. I tried to calm myself down. I thought, *Things are fine every day when I squeeze this bag, so if I squeeze this bag, things will be fine.* Still, the patient's chest failed to rise.

For a brief moment I imagined myself somewhere else, magically transported to another world without trouble. But the dream passed on when I heard the deepening pitch of the pulse oximeter tone. When a patient's oxygen level is normal, the pulse oximeter twitters with a high, merry pitch and sounds like a bird happily trilling on a branch. But as a patient's oxygen level falls, so, too, does the pitch, ominously, as though the bird were being slowly strangled. When I heard the change, my mind raced: *Why did I go down this path? You fool!*

"Suffocation!" The thought darted through my mind. The sound of the pulse oximeter grew distinct and menacing, a low and throbbing rumble, like approaching thunder. The craft of anesthesia sometimes consists of making oneself strongest at a certain point; one must choose a point of attack and concentrate one's forces there. I inserted the laryngoscope and lifted with all my strength, using both my arms, searching frantically for the windpipe. Still, I saw nothing. Panic took deeper root.

I made two more attempts at intubation. The patient's face flowed with blood and saliva. It felt to my fingers as though it were a stream of melting tar flowing toward the patient's chest. I tried the mask again. I held the mask so tightly against the patient's face that my hand started to cramp. The pain traveled up to the tense muscles of my forearm, but I endured it without so much as moving my fingers, so desperate was I to get even a smidgeon of air into the patient's lungs. Still, no air made its way in.

My mind was frozen. Everything was frozen now, except for my right hand, which just kept squeezing the bag.

Mournfully, I realized I had reached a major decision point, for unless the muscle relaxant wore off in the next minute, and the patient started to breathe again on his own, the patient would suffer serious brain damage or die. It is the most serious step in the career of any anesthesiologist: to tell a surgeon to perform a tracheotomy under emergency conditions, which, at the very least, will leave a permanent testament to the crisis in the form of an ugly scar on the patient's neck. Yet there may be no other way to get air into a patient before the muscle paralytic wears off.

I looked at the staff. The nurse's eyes were popping. The surgical tech's mouth was wide open. The surgeon was agitated. His resident assistant was pale. The moment of reckoning was at hand.

"Should I call another anesthesiologist to come help?" asked the nurse. I said nothing. "Yes, I'll go ahead and call," she panted with agitation. Deep down I knew it would accomplish nothing, because the other anesthesiologist would likely have the same problem I had. In the meantime, the patient would go that much longer without oxygen.

"I don't want to do a trach if I don't have to. Let's wait a couple more minutes. I bet the succinylcholine will wear off any second now," said the surgeon with pretended self-assurance. I said nothing.

I had known all during my training that this moment would come; yet I had always planned on having a serious conversation with myself about what I would do, and somehow the time to do so had vanished into thin air, like smoke escaping from a chimney. Nobody knew about this planned conversation but me, and even I hadn't thought about it very often, occasionally at night, during a bout of insomnia. Yet I had counted on it, and now it was too late; there was no more time.

My hair fell over my brow, and with my dirty palm I brushed it back, causing my cap to come off. I glanced at the blank, dying gaze of the patient's bloodshot eyes. Blood and saliva ran from the patient's mouth onto the pillow. I knew death was imminent; yet I deluded myself into agreeing with the nurse, thinking that the right thing to do was to wait for help, as well as with the surgeon, thinking that while we waited the patient would probably start to breathe again on his own. Hope against hope—the unreasonable hope of the panic-stricken mind. Then I thought about what people would say about me if they found out my patient needed a trach. It would be an embarrassing admission of failure on my part. Perhaps I should try intubating him one more time? Bit by bit, panic and fear were pushing me down a path, beaten out by many feet before me, ending in impenetrable underbrush where even the smartest doctor gets lost.

Suddenly, flashing through my head with the rapidity of lightning was the image of the attending who had told me as a resident that I would have to learn to eat shit and enjoy the taste of it, the one who had said that a doctor cannot be afraid. Next came the image of the cowboy-doctor who had called me a "chicken." *A doctor cannot fear what other people say when doing what he or she thinks is right*, I thought. Then came the image of Dr. C, the monkey-turned-ass who had kept trying to intubate a patient, almost killing her. *No, a doctor does more than just keep trying to intubate*, I thought. Then came the image of BSN, MSN, who had called the management of a medical crisis a "team activity" that demanded "input from all parties," who had talked like a senator, all while failing to produce the one thing that everyone wanted: a positive outcome. *No, in a crisis someone must take command*, I thought. Then followed the image of the patients who had tried to dictate their care to me—of the doctor's wife, in particular, who would have been furious to be left with a tracheotomy scar on her perfect neck. *Well, that's too bad*, I thought. *An imperfect plan put into action at the right time is better than a perfect one accomplished too late.*

My heart beat loud but evenly, driving through my body a new sense of concentrated energy. *Only to get air in!* I thought. The one idea possessed me. I stared at the surgeon and ordered him to perform the tracheotomy. The nurse seemed surprised. "What?" she asked. But the surgeon sensed my determination and jumped into action. Within thirty seconds the tracheotomy was in place. Air moved into the patient's lungs.

We strained our ears waiting for the pulse oximeter's pitch to rise in sweetness. Ten seconds of painful suspense. It did rise, slowly. After thirty seconds, it returned to normal. A happy, trilling chirp. So dear to the heart was the sound that all of us avidly listened without stirring, our faces still lime-white with residual fear.

The patient woke up and started breathing on his own five minutes later. He was fine and had suffered no brain damage. Five short minutes, and yet it might have made all the difference between a future life enjoying his children and grandchildren, and brain death.

But then the doubts returned. I kicked myself for having put the patient to sleep without a breathing tube in the first place. And I had regrets about his neck scar. My spirits had gone from being satisfied to being as foul and low as if I had been caught doing something awful. That night, I had a bad dream. I dreamed that I had paralyzed a patient with a muscle relaxant, and then, as I reached for the anesthesia bag to breathe for the patient, I discovered that my hands were too heavy to do so, as though they had been filled with lead. Then I saw that the bag itself was missing.

The patient turned blue while I looked on helplessly. I called out indistinctly in my sleep and tried to jump up.

The day after my near catastrophe a senior doctor approached me. I had never liked him very much. He was always a little cold and stiff. I feared he was going to berate me for what had happened. Instead, he said, "I heard what happened yesterday. Good job, doctor." Usually he addressed me by my first name, but this time he called me "doctor." That, plus his friendly tone, took me aback.

"But I blew it," I shrugged. "My patient needed a trach."

The senior doctor shook his head. "Being a doctor doesn't mean being perfect. All doctors make mistakes. And being a doctor isn't about knowing the most science or being the best at procedures. Being a doctor means knowing how to make decisions and take responsibility for them. It means admitting that you and everyone else in the room are on the wrong path, and getting them all back on the right path. It means giving a command and sticking to your guns. That's what you did, doctor. Good job," he said.

I was still a little confused, but I was coming around. He knew I was feeling better. He comfortably patted me on the back and said, "Don't worry. You know too much, you grow old too soon." Then he walked away. *What an enormous part of a person's nature is unknown to others*, I thought as I watched him pass out of sight.

In fact, I did feel better, much better. When I left for home that evening, I felt for the first time in my life that I was a doctor. The feeling was infinitely satisfying; it wound itself pleasantly around me. I forgot about the monotony of medical practice. I forgot about being so harried at work that I had missed lunch again. I forgot about the fights I had had over the years with other doctors, nurses, patients, and hospital administrators. At that moment nothing mattered to me anymore. I looked through the car window. In spite of the darkness, the air seemed to be shot through with moonlight; in spite of the slow traffic and loud city noises, nature seemed eager to be set free. Yes, I knew I was a doctor, and I knew what a doctor was, and I knew where I was going, and I knew why I was going there. My chest expanded, my heart pounded, and contentment raced at a gallop through my veins.

DEATH

I was in my last year of training. My patient was an eighty-year-old man with terminal cancer, congestive heart failure, and a bowel obstruction, now septic. In physiology, everything is coupled and connected, every organ system hangs, lies, touches, and rubs, one piece on another. This man's organ systems were collapsing. When I met him in the holding area he lacked the strength to speak, instead just gazing out onto the world with sorrowful eyes. We wheeled him into the operating room and moved him onto the table. I injected the drugs. Before losing consciousness, he looked up into my eyes, while I stared down into his. A flash of awareness seemed to register on the man's face. Each of us recognized the vital import of what was about to happen. Then a black, noiseless emptiness closed over the man, and the tie was broken.

More tumor had caused the bowel obstruction. The surgeon tried to de-bulk it. An hour into the case, the EKG alarm went off. Tall, wild, random markings tore the screen into jagged, angry pieces. A minute later, I heard the inexpressibly mournful tone of an EKG gone flatline. I watched the surgeon hovering above the man bring his clenched hands down on the patient's chest. CPR. The room heard the sickening scrunch of breaking ribs. The operating room team was unable to revive him.

I stared anxiously at the dead man's body. Through the blue mesh cap, I could see the patches of bald on the back of his head. I spotted the wrinkled arm with its blood pressure cuff still squeezing in a futile search for a blood pressure. I stared at the man's bloodless lips gleaming in the operating room lights, and the worn toenails.

In the dead "O" of his toothless mouth a savage groan was frozen stiff. I tried to convince myself that it was really astonishment, not horror, that lay on the man's face, that having just died he had seen the face of God. But his glassy eyes stared out with seemingly sorrowful pensiveness, and I realized that no one would look like that if they had seen God.

Sickness in a child evokes more sympathy than sickness in an old man, as an old man has already lived his life. But the appearance of death is as terrible in an old man as in a child. The mouth moves no more, the nose twitches no more—all this in someone who had once been dreaming, talking, and laughing.

We covered the man so as little of death as possible would peep out. A strange, hushed mood reigned in the room—the mood that comes at significant moments sensed by all, if not entirely understood by all.

I went back to the anesthesia lounge, sat down, and shut my eyes. It's not often that a person sees the life of another finish its long arc in his own hands. I thought about how the man had stared up into my face before losing consciousness. I somehow felt honored, having formed one of the two boundaries of the man's life. His first image may have been of the world before the age of the automobile; his last image had been of me. Factual details, but vital; they hold a life together. It was as if fate had been guiding the man toward me all these years, every event in his life moving him inexorably closer toward me, to its predestined endpoint. Still, I didn't really know the man. A beginning and end define a line, but not a life.

A patient death is a tragedy and never something that a doctor gets used to. Yet even as late as the 1970s, when a patient died under anesthesia, it was reportedly not uncommon for anesthesiologists to have said, "The patient took a bad anesthetic," or "It was God's will." Such doctors were distinguished by a certain emotional—no, not deafness, that would be too strong—by a certain emotional imprecision; it was as if some vaguely anxious thought about the dead patient had dawned on the threshold of their consciousness but didn't quite dawn. The attitude in those days seems to have been that sometimes an unexpected patient death comes just as it is, without any obligation for blame attached, or at least without any obligation to blame in any particularly cumbersome fashion. Today, of course, an unexpected patient death automatically triggers blame and a lawsuit. People no longer assume that death comes just as it is.

It's hard to comprehend the detached sensibility of that earlier era. For anesthesiologists of the past, maybe the fact that their patients were already asleep let them adjust more easily to the passage from life to death, given how they were already predisposed to accept death as a common occurrence. Frightful is the moment of passage from life to death—in an awake patient. The dying person falls or sputters or fights for air; there is a final struggle; and only afterward does the end come. Anesthetized patients, by contrast, are already still.

Yet this grudging acceptance of death seems to have existed beyond anesthesiology and even beyond medicine. Elderly people have told me stories of how family members died under anesthesia in the middle of the last century. When I ask for details, they confess ignorance, as no investigation was ever conducted. Growing angry on their behalf, I offer to review any old operating room records to see what went wrong. Instead of thanking me, these people stare at me quizzically and say, "Why bother? You can't change anything anyway. These things just happen." I assume the angry feeling in me is also inside them, absolutely invisible from the outside, but still there. Yet it is not there. To this day, in my effort to gauge the significance of their blunted feeling toward the death of a loved one, it is hard for me to know whether to pity or admire them.

I've never had a healthy patient die unexpectedly in the operating room. But I know that if such a thing happened, I would be numb with horror, with my own imaginings, and with what I would see as my own guilt, my guilt alone. Compared to anesthesiologists of the past, or at least anesthesiologists of legend, I would behave like a neurotic idiot. Colleagues of mine have admitted they would behave similarly. Perhaps the rarity of death in the operating room these days has sensitized doctors to the event. The death rate from anesthesia was 1 in 2,500 cases in the 1950s. Today it is 1 in 500,000 cases, even though far sicker patients are operated on now than before. A world where people rationalize an unexpected operating room death with the phrase "He took a bad anesthetic" has vanished forever into limbo.

I look upon my nervous anxiety toward death as a serious weakness in a doctor. Indeed, one reason I went into anesthesiology instead of surgery was that surgeons are usually responsible for breaking any bad news to family members. I once gave anesthesia to a teenage boy who had been rushed to the hospital with a gunshot wound to the head. He had bright red hair that fell to the ground when shaved off for surgery. Barely clinging to life even before the operation, he died afterward in the recovery room. When leaving the floor I saw a woman who must have been the boy's mother, waiting anxiously in the hall. She had the same red hair. Thankfully, I was spared from having to tell her the awful news.

This book is a journey of self-discovery. Over time I learned what a doctor is. But to this day, I have never really learned how to cope with patient death or to communicate a death to a family member. I consider it a failure on my part. That I have yet to be tested is no proof against this deficiency. It is not events or successes that produce good doctors, but rather a state of mind that can endow events with its own quality; a good doctor must possess a particular state of mind rather than trust to the recurrence of luck to keep its absence from being exposed.

My father had this necessary state of mind. Suffering usually passes through a doctor. He learns to ignore it so that he can work. But sometimes it catches on something inside and strongly affects him. My father was like that. He was quiet and sullen whenever a patient he liked and had been taking care of for years died. At such moments he preferred to be left alone in his study. While he eventually moved on, the deaths over time got to him, sometimes in odd ways. I think his obsession with tennis or travel, for example, came in part from the urge to seize hold of his life and not to put things on hold, given how life can vanish so quickly into thin air. Still, no matter where he went or what he did, he seemed to carry death on his back. Behind his happiness, somewhere, always lurked a haunting, undefined anxiety, of which he was never entirely free. Even at his happiest moments, there was a tinge of doubting sadness, as though he thought his happiness was not really justified. Living means remembering. My father told a lot of people they were dying. He told a lot of family members that their loved ones were dying. He saw a lot of death. That, to him, was part of being a doctor.

This grim acceptance of the facts of life is vital to the doctor's state of mind. A doctor must be able to witness death, to handle death, and to accept death. Even if death happens under his watch, he must be able to say, "Perhaps I acted unwisely; I might have been wrong, but I did my best," and then go back to work. I do not think I could do that. Indeed, when catastrophe looms in the operating room, I work feverishly to save my patient, not just for my patient's sake but also for my own. If a patient died by my own hand, I would be crushed. I'd probably quit medicine. I lack this vital ingredient of the good doctor. I lack a mature outlook on death.

This mature outlook is not the unique possession of the doctor, by the way. Why some people have it while others do not has always mystified me. As a teenager, while working as a hospital orderly, I saw my first dead body. It bothered me tremendously. One of the janitors saw this. Although largely uneducated, he gave me wiser counsel than anything I learned later on in medical school. He said, "Everyone is afraid of dead people. Only, if you work in a hospital, you have to tell yourself not to be afraid. And you can't act afraid. Sort of like giving yourself orders. And that's all that matters." Then he added, "But you're still afraid." He had the right outlook.

There is nothing constant in the world of medicine but sorrow. Death doesn't stop. No, death never stops for doctors, even for doctors who know what being a doctor means. It just haunts their souls and appears without invitation and absorbs their joys, their little human joys. Such is the construction of the world.

11

WHAT IS A DOCTOR?

A doctor is neither a scientist nor a technician nor a benefactor nor a jobholder. A doctor is a fighter. A doctor has spine. A doctor doesn't fear being called bad names. A doctor is flexible but sticks to his or her guns when necessary. A doctor is an authentic individual. A doctor has imagination and a sense of other people's lives. A doctor knows how to use the minds of others. A doctor commands, but also smoothes over controversies, motivates reluctant subordinates, and knows the limits of those subordinates. A doctor is not an elitist; he or she knows that even stupid people must have their say. A doctor has a passion for his or her profession, but recognizes the importance of other worlds beyond his or her profession. The doctor calmly assimilates other worlds, not just to broaden his or her consciousness but also to clear his or her mind. The doctor knows how to put the medical profession aside and take it up again. What is a doctor?

A doctor is a leader. These are the qualities of a leader.

A doctor's mind has successive coatings—science, technique, compassion, and instinct. A doctor is made of all these coatings. But at bottom he or she must be a leader. A sound doctor has his or her foundation deep in this inner coating. The rest are just the pediments and columns that rise up into the bright regions of the mind. If they form the only coatings, catastrophe looms. A scientist obsesses about rules; a technician obsesses about the craft of medicine; the benefactor obsesses about pleasing the patient; the jobholder obsesses about time off. Each gives rise to its own genre of medical catastrophe.

Without a doctor in command, the whole of medicine lacks an essential core, in the absence of which catastrophes occur. This is my argument. The catastrophes themselves are political in origin. Politics is about relationships, but at root it is about how people see their place in the world. Today, many doctors are unsure of their place because they do not know what a doctor is. Competing models vie for their attention, but each has a downside. The public hates the cold scientist; the doctor as technician is too easily emulated by non-MDs; the doctor as benefactor can barely make a living; the doctor as gentleman seems too elitist in a democratic age. There are even worse downsides—for patients—as each of these models carries with it the risk of catastrophe.

The confusion that doctors feel about their identities inevitably spawns real politics. The most important quality in a leader is that of being acknowledged as such. Today, doctors are not so acknowledged. Patients want to control medicine. So, too, do hospital administrators, bureaucrats, nurses, and insurance executives. With doctors confused about who they are, no one seems to be in control, and others want to step in and take control. Fighting ensues, putting the patient at risk. True, doctors still have power and say, but not enough to quell the fighting. The situation in medicine today is analogous to a country split by factions, where the dominant group represents only a little over half the voters. If the other groups feel anything like hatred for the leading group, the situation is dangerous. This is medicine today. Patient care proceeds in doubt and disagreement, as doctors lack the confidence of the other parties.

The doctors' confusion has spawned not only politics but also ideology. Patient activists push "rights" and "patient-centered care." Nurse activists push "team medicine." Administrators push "quality of care" and "accountable care." All these aspirational ideas have a noble purpose. But when taken to the extreme they raise the risk of catastrophe. Whenever people are required to act together, there must be a chief. By pushing doctors aside, these ideologies throw medical decision making into disarray. That disarray is often more the fault of the ideology's practitioners than the ideology itself, which should not surprise. Although reform movements are often necessary, the reformers themselves can be unattractive, obnoxious, fanatical people. Doctors complain about these people. And yet their very existence stems from the doctors' own identity confusion. Doctors have only themselves to blame for their coming into being.

Much attention has been paid in the last decade to catastrophes and near catastrophes in medicine. The bulk of that attention has been focused on physician error and how to correct for it. Drs. Atul Gawande and Peter Pronovost push checklists, time-outs, and protocols to address the problem. These modalities have real value. But at some point more protocols yield less return. They reach for the high-hanging fruit; they try to make an already rare medical catastrophe even more rare. They even turn counterproductive as medical personnel focus more on complying with the new protocols than on caring for patients.

Yet my purpose is not to belittle these important reforms but to call attention to an altogether different source of trouble. A doctor's judgment is often swayed by other side considerations that have nothing to do with medicine. It is not just error or forgetfulness that causes catastrophes but also politics. Many doctors today fear their colleagues; they fear their employers; they worry about crossing the nurses; they worry about antagonizing their patients; they even fear themselves. All this can cause catastrophe. Today, a parallel world of catastrophes rooted in politics sits alongside a world of catastrophe rooted in error.

The fix begins with the medical profession itself. The American Association of Medical Colleges predicts a shortage of a million doctors in the United States by 2025, with a third of that shortage in primary care.[1] To lessen that shortage, more medical schools are being built. The shortage is based on current models of doctoring—for example, the doctor as scientist, or technician, or caregiver. But if medical schools were to produce leaders, then the shortage would evaporate, as other professionals would take over the doctors' traditional roles, necessitating fewer doctors.

For example, the doctor-as-technician model has doctors performing most procedures and writing most prescriptions, and fighting nurses and other professionals to keep it that way. This notion once made sense. Decades ago, nurses were unevenly trained. Many drugs on formulary had a low therapeutic index, meaning the difference between a drug's therapeutic dose and its toxic dose was small, demanding a physician's education and experience to be prescribed safely. This is not the case today. Nurses are better trained. They must meet higher education standards. Drugs on formulary are much safer. Nurses and other professionals also have technology to help them, whether in the form of computers to assist in diagnosis and treatment or machines to help them safely perform small procedures. Moreover, when they do these procedures over and over again, they get good at them—even better than some doctors. Nurses and other non-MD professionals function well as highly skilled technicians.

None of this should threaten doctors who see themselves as leaders, for this is what doctors must become. Being technicians is no longer how doctors add value. Doctors add value through supervising, governing, and coordinating, whether in the care of a single patient or a large demographic group. They legitimate a patient plan and give it binding force, not just for the obvious reason that they give the orders but also because their broad consciousness is a unique source of power. In the future, when a conflict arises between parties in a patient's care or during a medical crisis, doctors will be presumed to have all the facts, to be supplied with the best available intelligence of all kinds, and to have the diplomatic skills needed to get all the parties on the same track. This will make doctors the real arbiters among the many well-thought-out therapeutic options presented to them by nurses, computers, and robots.

Such a system requires fewer doctors, especially in primary care, where much of the physician shortage is expected. The days of doctors fighting nurses over every inch of turf must end. Doctors must cede more of their turf. Health care costs alone demand this. True, this plan works less well in surgery than in medicine. Surgery, by definition, is procedure focused, and the tight connection between a surgeon's advanced cognitive skills and his or her procedural skills forestalls a serious off-loading of technical tasks onto nurses and computers. Indeed, a fundamental divide once existed between medicine and surgery, one that waned during the twentieth century, but one that will likely return for the next few decades—at least until robots become as proficient as computers. When that happens, non-MDs armed with robots may be as useful as non-MDs armed with computers. Still, the doctors' leadership role will remain vital.

This change should excite doctors, not scare them. The natural tendency of technicians is to do more of the same, which is dull. Doctors who are leaders will move beyond such thinking. Instead, they will have an overall view of everything that is going on in the patient care setting. Even if they have relatively less power over day-to-day patient matters, doctors will be thought to have the best knowledge of the entire situation. People will tend to believe in them. They will enjoy more respect. Their days will grow less monotonous. It is a work of art to lead people, and as the routine technical side of doctoring is offloaded, doctors will enjoy a higher share of interesting work. For nurses and other non-MDs, work will expand to include technical and decision-making responsibilities that have largely been denied to them. For the health care system as a whole, fewer doctors will be needed as nurses and other non-MD professionals, computers, and robots fill roles that doctors vacate.

This plan will also reduce the risk of medical catastrophe. Catastrophe arises from disorder and conflict as doctors, nurses, administrators, regulators, and patients fight one another. They fight because, at root, they don't know where they stand. They don't know who has the right to command and who must obey. They rebel in their hearts against what they perceive to be an unjust usurpation of their own prerogatives. A secret internal warfare pervades the entire field, with patients suffering most of all. By transforming doctors into leaders, the other players in medicine, including patients, will enjoy stable turf they can control, giving them a sense of dignity and the feeling of productive activity. The result will be a safer system for patients, analogous to what prevailed in my father and grandfather's era, when all the players in medicine lived together in order and peace.

Some doctors will disagree with this plan. They want to resurrect the old, for which they pine. They want to put the pieces back together and re-create the vision of doctoring that prevailed during much of the twentieth century—part scientist, part technician, part benefactor, and part gentleman. However, this dream is not only impossible and undesirable but also misplaced. That vision itself was the product of erroneous thinking, made possible by a sudden explosion in scientific knowledge during the second half of the nineteenth century, and the subsequent doctors' monopoly on that knowledge during the first half of the twentieth century. It was a short moment in history, when doctors were scientists and technicians first. In the millennium before, most doctors added value to medicine not as scientists or technicians or benefactors but as leaders.

Medical historian Nancy Siraisi's account of the physician Bartholomeus managing the care of Peter the Venerable in the twelfth century provides an example.[2] Although a layman, Peter was confident in his medical knowledge. During a bout of flu-like symptoms he accepted the advice of local caregivers and postponed his routine bloodletting, since they told him he risked losing his voice if he underwent the procedure. A few months later, he went ahead with the bloodletting, thinking his caregivers wrong. Still, his flu-like symptoms persisted. And he lost his voice.

His caregivers then recommended hot and moist remedies. But the well-educated Peter disagreed. According to his reading, hot and dry remedies were called for. Frustrated with his care, he wrote to Bartholomeus, who, with artful diplomacy, managed the ticklish situation. Bartholomeus generally agreed with the local caregivers but tactfully avoided directly contradicting Peter, so as not to antagonize any of the parties involved. He also used his extra knowledge to dress up the routine therapies prescribed by the local caregivers and lend them weight, at least in Peter's mind. By today's standards, Bartholomeus was a poor scientist and technician; yet he was the consummate leader, resolving a conflict between a headstrong patient and the caregivers the patient had lost faith in, while steering the patient toward what professional medicine at the time believed to be right course.

For eighty years, American doctors saw themselves as a mixture of scientist, technician, benefactor, and gentleman. For two thousand years before that, doctors saw themselves as leaders. The latter vision wins by weight alone. A person may be wrong, and so may several generations, but humanity rarely makes mistakes.

Medicine has changed, although it is easier to see this now, thirty years after most of the events in this book occurred, and when the change actually began. For older doctors, medicine did not change especially fast, but gradually medical practice has become strange and unfamiliar to them. Many of them embrace the new ways unwillingly, clumsily, and halfheartedly. In fact, in their hearts they do not accept the new system, and instead have contempt for it. Never surrendering fully, they only pretend they have. Younger doctors never knew the old way. Still, some of them have heard legends, and when they encounter the reality of medical practice rather than the charmed life they had imagined, they are disappointed. They go from a time in their lives when they can neither think about evil nor believe in its existence to their first years of practice, when they work against the system and grow cynical and frustrated. Day after day goes by in battling against the obstinacy of some official or repairing the blunders of a fool. They imagine nothing can be done; to have an immense plan for health care would be useless, and even after just a few years in practice they know it.

To cause people to be disgusted by their own work is a serious error on the part of organized medicine. What could be more natural than doctors liking what they do? But many of them don't like it.

What bothers many doctors is the loss of their independence. They dislike being employed, by whatever institution, although they do like having their malpractice insurance paid for by an institution, as well as having an institution's clerks do their billing. Lawyers have analogous complaints. They like the security and convenience of employment, but they resent their loss of autonomy. For both groups, there has been a change. In the nineteenth century, law and medicine were typically referred to as the "free professions" because lawyers or doctors could set up shop anywhere and be their own bosses. Today, law and medicine remain professions, but they are increasingly less free, with lawyers and doctors working as dependent, salaried employees.

Still, such griping will probably wane over the years. When I started my training, most medical students aspired to be small businesspeople and run their own shops, a mentality out of sync with employed work. Today's students seem less interested in being businesspeople.

Yet even if most doctors grow comfortable with being employed, dependent employment raises the risk of medical catastrophe. Sometimes doctors feel trapped between employers who demand one course of action and patients who insist on another. They feel barred from choosing what they think is the wisest course of action. The patient suffers.

The risk of catastrophe is so great that this author, who has always supported private practice medicine, is tempted to choose national health insurance as the second option rather than the emerging model of dependent employment in the private sector. Although Medicare-for-all would pay doctors less, doctors would keep much of their autonomy, at least in theory. Compare this with the plight of an employed physician who recently complained to me that she couldn't even choose her own receptionist. The company that employs her does the hiring and firing, and when it hired someone who was nasty to her patients, causing many of them to leave, there was nothing she could do. Then again, the benefits of Medicare-for-all are only theoretical. In reality, Medicare pays too little to allow most independent doctors' offices to survive. In addition, Medicare's regulators can be as intrusive as private-sector bosses—for example, by fighting with physicians over what drug they can prescribe. Neither the second option nor the third fixes the problem.

Doctors today find themselves in a difficult situation. Still, the blame for their situation lies not with government or corporate America but with the doctors themselves. When doctors ceased to be leaders, they opened themselves up to being employed, and not just because their technical approach to medicine lent itself to an employment model. They also refused to make the tough decisions about who would get care that government and corporate America now make. If I were a corporate executive confronting a physician whining about his or her loss of autonomy, I would yell right back at that physician:

"You know why corporate America took over medicine? It's because we provided a solution to the doctors' spinelessness. Everyone knows that unlimited high-quality medical care is a pipedream for now. Tough decisions have to be made, gut-wrenching decisions. Decisions that may cost some people their lives! And who's going to make them? Who's going to say, 'Sorry, you still want something from life, but you can't have it, because there's not enough money'? Do you want government making those decisions? Everyone's afraid of government; even the politicians worry about getting too involved. Do you want 'the people' making these decisions? Ah, yes, 'the people,' always the people. Why, they're the source of all this trouble, whipped up by those pie-in-the-sky activists, those seekers of truth, those fighters for justice, those representatives of the insulted and the injured who peddle ridiculous expectations about health care being a right, but who know nothing about how to run a business. 'The people' are in no position to make these decisions. And so everyone hoped the doctors would make them—those wise, thoughtful professionals, those learned men and women gifted with nuance and subtlety. Everyone secretly hoped the doctors would make the hard decisions, although no one said so in public, since the notion of health care as a universal right was still official ideology. But you know what the doctors did? They balked, the little cowards! We had counted on them to take the power, to be wise and judicious fathers, but they were too afraid! They said, 'We don't have the stomach for this. Our forefathers may have, but we're different. Our consciences, our precious consciences . . . why, we have to deal with patients face to face! Find a way to spread the burden of deciding, so that the consequences won't fall on any one of us individually.' And in response to that pathetic, weak-kneed plea, corporate American's health care bureaucracy was born: layers and layers of utilization review specialists, insurance regulators, practitioners, secretaries, and switchboard operators, all playing their role in gumming up the process, keeping people from getting care, holding down costs, and each one, along with the doctors taking for themselves a tiny slice of the blame for a patient's death—not enough to keep anyone awake at night with a bad conscience but enough to do what's necessary to keep the system solvent."

This is the ugly truth. In an environment of sparse resources and high demand, corporate America and government took over when doctors abdicated the position they held in days when health care was considered a "privilege" rather than a "right." As the final arbiters of who would get care, doctors once carried a heavy burden. By deciding to treat someone based on ability to pay, doctors held the power of life and death. Doctors no longer play this leadership role, and they would not want it back if offered to them. The public also prefers it this way. Doctors are human beings, and for a human being to be complicit in a decision about resources that causes another person's death is called "murder." Alternatively, when an institution makes such decisions, the human element disappears. Bad outcomes arise from the "system's limitations." Although people compose a system, the public conveniently overlooks the fact that a system is composed of people.

Today's system no longer asks doctors to make decisions about resources. Yet it still demands leadership from doctors, even employed doctors, to prevent catastrophes. Such leadership requires protections for doctors. In theory, leaders shouldn't need protections. Leaders are fearless. They stand firm. They do not put their pleasures above their responsibilities. But let's be honest: most doctors aren't leaders. They went into medicine to enjoy interesting work, make a good living, and do something worthwhile for humanity in the process. And so most doctors are not fearless. To make the right decisions for patients, they need protection from fear. I suggest a tenure system for employed physicians, analogous to what reigns in academia: after five years an employed physician enjoys more job security, so that he or she feels less afraid when making tough decisions that benefit patients.

The doctor as leader is a vision and, for the time being, a fantasy. Yet if I were asked what is the one thing missing from medicine today, causing doctors to hate their work and patients to complain about their care, I would say it is the disappearance of fantasy from medicine. The history of American medicine is worth separating into fact and dream. This book focuses on fact. Yet there is something in the dream that still touches patients and those who care for them, and remains worthwhile because it resonates with them as much as fact does: the dream of people wholly absorbed in a struggle to save a person's life, fused within a collective group and yet still separate parts. It was the dream of my father and grandfather's eras, when doctors and their spouses, nurses, Catholic sisters, and administrators each played their own special role in the drama, replete with special uniforms, giving the hospital the feel of a magic country, and the experience of being sick almost an inexpressible charm. Patients today cling to this legend and are loath to give it up. In their bewildered state they search in their imaginations for something to comfort them while ill, and they mix the realities of their caregivers with a little bit of fairy tale.

The dream brings to mind a symphony, where different instruments that might otherwise play a separate melody come together to create a perfectly harmonized hymn. Perhaps the music today is outdated, but it was beautiful, and who doesn't love beauty? A dying patient would rather die in his sleep, but if he can't, how much better to fall unconscious with that tender, beautiful music in his ears; how much better to die to that music than to do so in a cacophonous modern facility staffed by anonymous "providers"?

If a terminally ill patient once dreamed of dying to that music, the doctor, the nurse, the doctor's spouse, and the Catholic sister once lived for it. Amid that great intangible melody, these caregivers not only fantasized about each other *but also fantasized about themselves*, as each had something special about them, each had something the others could admire but not share in. Perhaps that special ingredient was an unattainable ideal—a legend in dreams that could never become a legend in fact—but through it, each person working in the hospital imagined his or her life unrolling itself on a grand, almost mythical level. How proud to be the doctor, the nurse, or the Catholic sister of legend! How proud to do things with ceremony, gravity, drama, and solemnity! How wonderful to fire another's imagination—and one's own! How wonderful to be special, honored, respected, and even worshipped! And how much better to be a part of a magnificent symphony than to be a generic "provider" in a modern facility, humming a stupid tune or, worse, creating a clamor through discord, for what unique passions and excitement could a provider possibly have with which to create music? The provider is like everyone else. He or she dresses like all the other providers; he or she has the same strengths, the same worries, and the same weaknesses as the other providers. The new order in health care may be efficient. It is certainly more advanced than in my father and grandfather's time. But there are no distinctive parts to the orchestra, and so there is no symphony. None of its music stirs the blood.

Change begins with doctors. Once they change, the rest of medicine will fall into place and the music will begin again. Doctors must become leaders.

NOTES

I. THE POLITICS OF A CATASTROPHE

1. Barron Lerner, "A Case That Shook Medicine," *Washington Post*, November 28, 2006.

2. IMPATIENCE AND THE URGE TO BE MACHO

1. Roni Rabin, "You're on the Clock: Doctors Rush Patients out the Door," *USA Today*, April 20, 2014.

3. THE TRAP OF OVERSPECIALIZATION

1. George Weisz, *Divide and Conquer: A Comparative History of Medical Specialization* (New York: Oxford University Press, 2005), 138–39, 145, 197, 231, 249.

2. "2014 Survey of America's Physicians: Practice Patterns and Perspectives," The Physicians Foundation, September 16, 2014, accessed April 1, 2016, http://www.physiciansfoundation.org/news/survey-of-20000-us-physicians-shows-80-of-doctors-are-over-extended-or-at.

4. WHEN NO ONE IS IN COMMAND

1. Bachelor of Science in Nursing and Master of Science in Nursing.
2. Dilation (of the cervix) and curettage (scraping) of the uterus.

5. WHEN PATIENTS BECOME CONSUMERS

1. Kristine Crane, "Should You 'Friend' Your Doctor?" *U.S. News and World Report*, May 22, 2014.
2. In my own practice, I once had a mother panic when her child coughed and sputtered while going under anesthesia. The mother refused to leave the room, requiring the nurses to attend to her, which delayed us in our efforts to help her child.
3. Donald Berwick, "Stepping into Power, Shedding Your White Coat" (graduation speech at Yale Medical School commencement ceremony, May 24, 2010).
4. Dorothy Wertz et al., "Has Patient Autonomy Gone Too Far?" *American Journal of Bioethics* 2, no. 4 (2002): 1–25.
5. Donald Berwick, "What 'Patient-Centered' Should Mean: Confessions of an Extremist," *Health Affairs* 28, no. 4 (July/August 2009): w555–w565.

6. A TALE OF TWO OFFICES

1. Now Medstar Washington Hospital Center.
2. For further discussion of these schools, see Ronald W. Dworkin, "Reimagining the Doctor," *National Affairs* 18 (Winter 2014): 63–77.
3. See Melnick Medical Museum, "1930 Doctor's Office," accessed April 16, 2016, https://melnickmedicalmuseum.com/exhibits/doctors-and-dentists-offices/.
4. Now the Armed Forces Retirement Home.

7. WHEN DOCTORS LOSE CONTROL OF THEIR OWN PERSONALITIES

1. Sanford Brown, *Getting into Medical School* (New York: Barron's Educational Series, 1997), 7.

2. Kenneth Ludmerer, "Instilling Professionalism in Medical Education," *JAMA* 282, no. 9 (1999): 881.

3. See *Initiative to Transform Medical Education*, the final report of the 2007 conference of the American Medical Association, accessed April 10, 2016, http://med2.uc.edu/Libraries/Medical_Education_Documents/AMA_ITME_Project.sflb.ashx.

4. See *Report of the Council on Medical Education*, American Medical Association, accessed April 16, 2016, http://www.ama-assn.org/assets/meeting/2011a/tab-ref-comm-c-addendum.pdf.

5. Veritas Prep, "Medical Schools Value Personal Qualities of Applicants," *U.S. News and World Report*, January 16, 2012.

6. Brian Joondeph, "Politically Correct Medical Schools," *Washington Examiner*, June 18, 2015.

7. William Whyte, *The Organization Man* (New York: Anchor Books, 1957), 134.

8. WHEN DOCTORS LOSE CONTROL OF THEIR OWN RULES

1. Richard Baumgarten, "Spinal Anesthesia Research: Let's Not Be Hasty," in "Letters to the Editor" Section, *Anesthesia and Analgesia* 105, no. 6 (December 2007): 1862.

2. See, for example, Atul Gawande, *The Checklist Manifesto* (New York: Metropolitan Books, 2009), and Peter Pronovost and Eric Vohr, *Safe Patients, Smart Hospitals* (New York: Hudson Street Press, 2010).

3. In a placenta previa, the placenta covers the opening of the birth canal and risks rupture during delivery.

9. THE PROBLEM OF GOING PART-TIME AND WHEN TO RETIRE

1. AMGA/Cejka Search 2011 Physician Retention Survey, cited in Dike Drummond, "Part Time Doctor: Physician Schedule Flexibility and the New Normal," *The Happy MD* (blog), accessed April 16, 2016, http://www.thehappymd.com/blog/bid/290765/Part-Time-Doctor-Physician-Schedule-Flexibility-and-the-New-Normal.

2. Robert Grossman and Steven Abramson, "Wanted: A Three-Year Medical Degree," *Wall Street Journal*, February 17, 2016.

3. "2014 Survey of America's Physicians," The Physicians Foundation, survey conducted by Merritt Hawkins, 2014, accessed on April 16, 2016, http://www.physiciansfoundation.org/uploads/default/2014_Physicians_Foundation_Biennial_Physician_Survey_Report.pdf.

11. WHAT IS A DOCTOR?

1. "Physician Supply and Demand through 2025: Key Findings," American Association of Medical Colleges, 2015 Report, accessed April 16, 2016, https://www.aamc.org/download/426260/data/physiciansupplyanddemandthrough2025keyfindings.pdf.

2. Nancy Siraisi, *Medieval and Early Renaissance Medicine* (Chicago: University of Chicago Press, 1990), 115.

BIBLIOGRAPHY

Baumgarten, Richard. "Spinal Anesthesia Research: Let's Not Be Hasty." In "Letters to the Editor" Section, *Anesthesia and Analgesia* 105, no. 6 (December 2007).

Berwick, Donald. "What 'Patient-Centered' Should Mean: Confessions of an Extremist." *Health Affairs* 28, no. 4 (July/August 2009): w555–w565.

Brown, Sanford. *Getting into Medical School.* New York: Barron's Educational Series, 1997.

Dworkin, Ronald W. "Re-imagining the Doctor." *National Affairs* 18 (Winter 2014): 63–77.

Gawande, Atul. *The Checklist Manifesto.* New York: Metropolitan Books, 2009.

Janvier, W. Ed, et al. *The Story of Garfield Memorial Hospital: 1881–1951.* Washington, DC: Washington College Press, 1951.

Ludmerer, Kenneth. "Instilling Professionalism in Medical Education." *JAMA* 282, no. 9 (1999): 881–82.

Pronovost, Peter, and Eric Vohr. *Safe Patients, Smart Hospitals.* New York: Hudson Street Press, 2010.

Riesman, David. *The Lonely Crowd.* New Haven, CT: Yale University Press, 1950.

Siraisi, Nancy. *Medieval and Early Renaissance Medicine.* Chicago: University of Chicago Press, 1990.

Weisz, George. *Divide and Conquer: A Comparative History of Medical Specialization.* New York: Oxford University Press, 2005.

Wertz, Dorothy, et al. "Has Patient Autonomy Gone Too Far?" *American Journal of Bioethics* 2, no. 4 (2002): 1–25.

Whyte, William. *The Organization Man.* New York: Anchor Books, 1957.

ABOUT THE AUTHOR

Ronald W. Dworkin, MD, works as an anesthesiologist while also teaching political philosophy in the George Washington University Honors Program. His essays on medicine, and on American culture and politics, have appeared in such publications as the *Wall Street Journal*, *National Affairs*, *Policy Review*, *The New Atlantis*, and *The Public Interest*. He lives in Maryland.